NUTRITION and FITNESS

50 Lessons and Exercises

Helen J. Miller

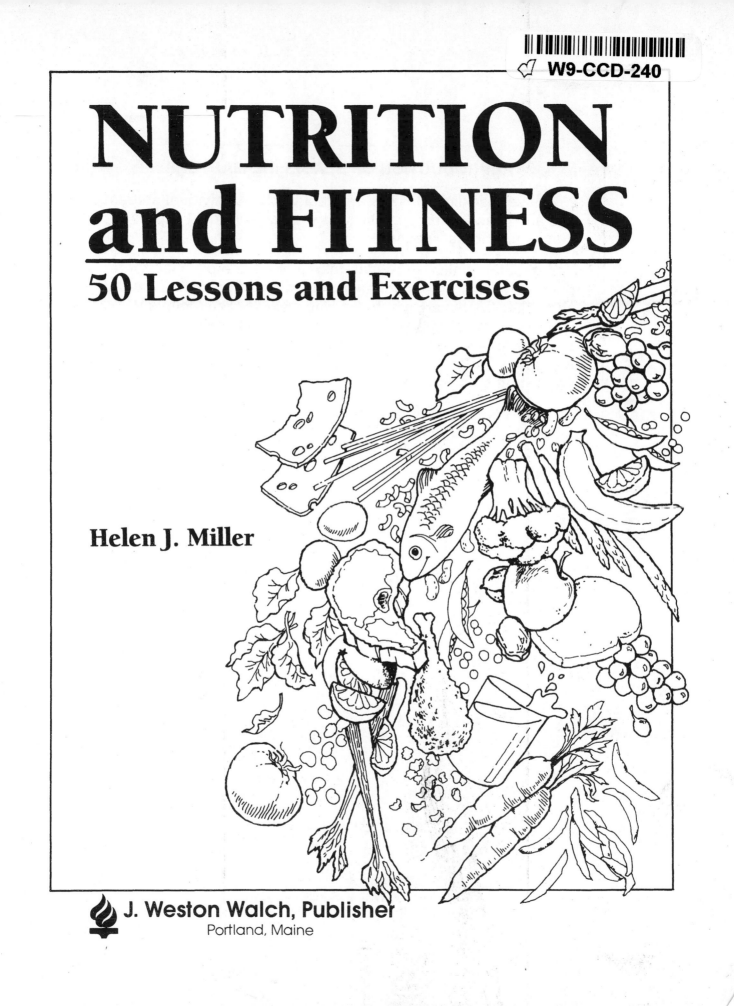

J. Weston Walch, Publisher

Portland, Maine

ISBN 0-8251-1616-3

1   2   3   4   5   6   7   8   9   10

Copyright © 1989
J. Weston Walch, Publisher
P.O. Box 658 • Portland, Maine 04104-0658

Printed in the United States of America

Acknowledgment

I wish to thank the Penn State Nutrition Center, in particular Faith L. Davies for her conscientious reviewing of this material.

Contents

REPRODUCIBLE MASTERS

Part I: *Individual Components of Nutrition*

Part II: *Putting the Components Together*

Section A: *Putting the Components Together to Eat Well*

Section B: *Putting the Components Together to Maintain an Ideal Weight*

Section C: *Putting the Components Together to Be a Wise Consumer*

Part III: *Evaluation of Knowledge and Attitudes*

Appendices

Introduction

Nutrition research, nutrition knowledge, and interest in nutrition have been increasing rapidly. Students are more interested in nutrition than they have been in the past. These worksheets have been designed to highlight current nutrition knowledge, beyond the basic four food groups, and to help students increase their understanding of current nutrition-related issues. The worksheets will provide activities that will help students learn the information and develop the skills needed to choose healthier diets for themselves and their families.

I have found that students who are active in athletics and those who are concerned about physical fitness are the students who are most interested in nutrition. Therefore, I have tried to emphasize, whenever possible, the relationship between nutrition and physical fitness. Since the nutrition needs of active teens are not too different from other, less-active teens, all students can benefit from this information.

Even the simplest meal or snack is a combination of nutrients and should be chosen to meet the complex nutritional needs of the person eating it. Thus, it seems appropriate to start teaching nutrition by introducing the individual parts of nutrition, the nutrients, and then work up to the skills needed to put the nutrients together into meals and diets.

Following this philosophy, I have divided these worksheets into these three parts.

Part I: *Individual Components of Nutrition*

This section includes activities to help students understand what is currently known about the nutrients and related matters. The relationship of nutrients to health is emphasized. When these individual topics are mastered, the students will have the tools to apply nutrition knowledge to the complexities of choosing foods that meet daily needs.

Part II: *Putting the Components Together*

With an understanding of the basics of nutrition, the students should be able to apply this knowledge to the selection of a healthy diet.

Section A

Activities in Section A are designed to help students evaluate daily eating situations. Students should be able to assimilate the best advice to choose healthy diets.

x   Nutrition and Fitness

Section B

Activities in Section B help the students apply nutrition knowledge to weight control, which is an area of interest to almost everyone. Statistics tell us that 75% of 19-year-old females admit to having been on a diet to lose weight. Wrestlers and gymnasts are constantly watching their weight. Weight control is also a popular topic for adults. Manufacturers advertise "lite" products. The media conveys the latest ways to slim down. Nutrition students need to discern information about weight control.

Section C

The popularity of nutrition has not been overlooked by business. Section C activities are designed to help students become wiser consumers of nutrition-related items.

Part III: *Evaluation of Knowledge and Attitudes*

The evaluation devices in this section may be used either as pretests to determine strengths and weaknesses, or as posttests to evaluate knowledge acquired.

Sources of Information

American Diabetes Association, Inc. Diabetes Information Service Center, 1660 Duke Street, Alexandria, VA 22314. Telephone: (800) ADA–DISC

The American Dietetic Association. 430 North Michigan Avenue, Chicago, IL 60611. Telephone: (312) 280–5000

American Heart Association. National Center, 7320 Greenville Avenue, Dallas, TX 75231.

Kowtaluk, Helen. *Discovering Nutrition.* Chas. A. Bennett Co., Inc., Peoria, IL 61615.

Food and Nutrition Information Center (FNIC), National Agricultural Library, Room 304, Beltsville, MD 20705. Telephone: (301) 344–3719

National Dairy Council. 6300 N. River Road, Rosemont, IL 60018-4233.

Hamilton, E., E. Whitney, and F. Sizer. *Nutrition: Concepts and Controversies.* 4th ed. 1987. West Publishing Co., 50 West Kellogg Blvd., P.O. Box 43526, St. Paul, MN 55164-0526. $39.00

Penn State Nutrition Center. Benedict House, Penn State University, University Park, PA 16802. Telephone: (814) 865–6323

United States Department of Agriculture. Human Nutrition Information Service, Room 325A, Federal Building, Hyattsville, MD 20782.

1. Protein Sources: Complete and Incomplete

Human beings need to eat protein that provides all the amino acids that cannot be produced by the body. Proteins that provide all the essential amino acids are known as complete proteins. These proteins come from animals. Plants also contain protein. No one plant protein has all the essential amino acids, so plant proteins are known as incomplete proteins.

Directions: This a list of foods that are all good sources of protein. Indicate which come from an <u>A</u>nimal source and contain <u>C</u>omplete proteins [AC] and which come from a <u>P</u>lant source and contain <u>I</u>ncomplete proteins [PI].

	Animal or Plant? A/P	Complete or Incomplete? C/I		Animal or Plant? A/P	Complete or Incomplete? C/I
1. Dried beans	P	I	16. Chicken	A	C
2. Milk	A	C	17. Cheese	A	C
3. Haddock	A	C	18. Cashews	P	I
4. Tuna	A	C	19. Tofu	P	I
5. Eggs	A	C	20. Lentils	P	I
6. Peanut butter	P	I	21. Pork	A	C
7. Bread	P	I	22. Turkey	A	C
8. Cereal	P	I	23. Chick-peas	P	I
9. Hamburger	A	C	24. Tortilla	P	I
10. Soybeans	P	I	25. Noodles	P	I
11. Wheat germ	P	I	26. Rice	P	I
12. Beef	A	C	27. Meatballs	A	C
13. Peas	P	I	28. Roll	P	I
14. Peanuts	A	I	29. Macaroni	P	I
15. Pasta	A	I	30. Black beans	P	I

Combining an incomplete plant protein with a small amount of complete animal protein provides food containing excellent protein. This combining of plant and animal protein also increases the variety in our diets while it usually decreases the amount of saturated fat in the diet.

Challenge: See how many plant-animal combinations you can make from the above list. You can use combinations that are familiar to you, such as a peanut butter sandwich and a glass of milk. To really increase your list, you can find combinations that may be better known in other parts of the world, such as fried rice with egg. Be sure to indicate the protein-rich ingredients and tell if they are plant or animal. *Example:* peanut butter and bread [PI], milk [AC] or rice [PI], egg [AC].

Name _____ Date _____

2. Complementary Proteins

The protein in egg white is considered nearly perfect because it contains 100% of all eight essential amino acids. In this diagram, four of the essential amino acids are represented by spokes.

T = Tryptophane

L = Lysine

I = Isoleucine

M = Methionine

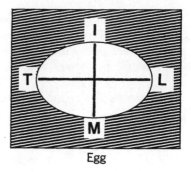

Egg

Plant proteins, as shown in the diagrams below, do not contain all the essential amino acids. That is why they are known as incomplete proteins.

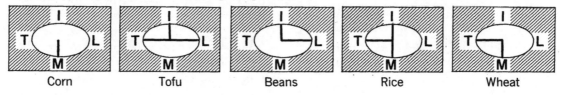

Corn   Tofu   Beans   Rice   Wheat

By combining plant proteins that complement each other, people all over the world have made dishes that provide very high-quality protein.

A. Directions: On each blank circle, draw the spokes to represent the amino acids present in the ingredients found in the dish listed under the circle.

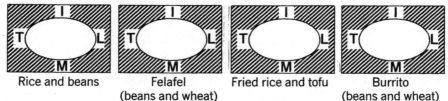

Rice and beans   Felafel   Fried rice and tofu   Burrito
             (beans and wheat)   (beans and wheat)

B. Directions: Now that you understand how these combinations work, create your own combinations. Be sure to identify the ingredients you use.

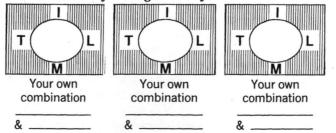

Your own   Your own   Your own
combination   combination   combination

_____   _____   _____
& _____   & _____   & _____

Directions: Answer these questions on the back of this sheet.

1. Do any of your combinations have missing essential amino acids? If they do, what could be eaten with these dishes to provide the missing amino acids?

2. What happens if you do not eat all eight essential amino acids within 24 hours?

3. Why would people choose to eat incomplete plant proteins instead of complete animal proteins?

        2   *Nutrition and Fitness*

3. How Much Protein Is Enough?

A. **Directions:** From the list below (or a more complete list from your teacher), choose foods to represent the amount of protein-rich foods you eat in a typical day. Add up the amount of grams of protein you eat in an average day.

Food	Amt.	Protein (g)	Food	Amt.	Protein (g)	Food	Amt.	Protein (g)
Milk	1 cup	8	Cheese	1 oz	7	Fish	1 oz	7
Poultry	1 oz	7	Bread	1 slice	2	Egg	1 large	7
Cereals	1 cup	4	Pizza	1 slice	15	Fruit	1 large	2
Vegetables	1 cup	2	Beef stew	1 cup	16	Spaghetti/		
Taco, beef	1	9	Hamburger	3 oz	21	meatballs	1 cup	19
Baked beans	1 cup	15	Milk shake	10 oz	11	Steak	3 oz	22
Peanut butter	1 tbsp	5	Chili	1 cup	26	Ice cream	1 cup	5
Enchilada	1	20	Macaroni and			Chop suey	1 cup	26
Lean meat	1 oz	7	cheese	1 cup	17	Hot dog	1	5

Total protein eaten on an average day is _____ grams.

How much protein do I need each day?

Each day a teenage girl will need about 46 grams of protein, a teenage boy about 56 grams. Very active growing teens, in training for a sport, and weighing 150 pounds would not need more than 68 grams of protein each day.

B. **Directions:** Compare the amount of protein you normally *eat* each day to the amount of protein you *need* each day. Considering the fact that we allowed more than enough protein per day to cover all needs, including athletic training and growth, what is your opinion about the necessity for you to eat extra protein-rich foods and/or to take protein supplements?

What happens to extra protein eaten?

C. **Directions:** Each gram of protein eaten provides 4 calories (the same as carbohydrate). Calculate how many calories were in the protein you ate for one day.

_____ grams of protein I ate

×   4   (calories in one gram of protein)

= _____ calories from protein

Each gram of extra protein provides extra calories. The body stores extra calories as fat. What does this tell us will happen to extra calories eaten as protein?

4. Fats

Directions: Except for one item, all the items in each problem are related to a single fact about or characteristic of fats. Your job is to determine the relationship, give the category its correct title, and then cross out the item that does not fit in that category. For example, all the items except one in the first problem are related to fat because they are fat-soluble vitamins. Vitamin B would be crossed out because it is a water-soluble vitamin. Refer to your textbook or another source, if you need to.

Titles you will use are: Low-Fat Grain Products, Low-Fat Desserts, Low-Saturated-fat Main Dishes, High-Fat Meats, Types of Fat, Polyunsaturated Oils, Monounsaturated Fats, Saturated Fats, Why Fat Is Essential, and Fat-Soluble Vitamins.

Title #1 _____
1. Vitamin A   Vitamin B   Vitamin D   Vitamin E   Vitamin K

Title #2 _____
2. Saturated   Monounsaturated   Polyunsaturated   Cholesterol

Title #3 _____
3. Cream   Cheese   Margarine   Ice cream   Butter

Title #4 _____
4. Olive oil   Popeye   Peanut oil   Margarine   Shortening

Title #5 _____
5. Coconut   Corn   Sunflower   Safflower   Cottonseed

Title #6 _____
6. Carry vitamins   Supply energy   Give flavor   Cushion organs   Give fiber

Title #7 _____
7. Roast beef   Hamburger   Broiled halibut   Ham   Pork chop

Title #8 _____
8. Low-fat yogurt   Ice milk   Sherbet   Chocolate cake   Angel food cake

Title #9 _____
9. Macaroni and cheese   Tuna salad   Dried beans   Steamed crabs   Roasted chicken

Title #10 _____
10. Shredded wheat   Rice   Doughnut   Bread   Bagel

Answer the following questions on a separate sheet of paper or on the back of this sheet.

11. What is the difference in the amount of calories in different types of fats?

12. Why is it recommended that we reduce the amount of total fat, saturated fat, and cholesterol that we eat?

Name _____ Date _____

5. What Is It?

It's a fatlike substance but it's not a fat.

Our bodies need it but we don't need to eat it.

Directions: Write the correct word beside each clue below. You may need to refer to your textbook or another source for some of the words. When you have finished, the circled letters will answer the question, "What Is It?"

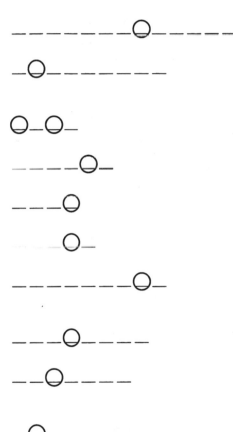

1. High blood levels of it contribute to the development of this condition which is a type of hardening of the arteries.

2. This person can tell you if you should not eat it.

3. It is found in foods with animal fats but not in this liquid fat from plants.

4. Heart disease is America's number one _____.

5. The yolks of these contain large amounts of it.

6. To control your intake of it, limit your use of organ _____.

7. Eating this type of fat tends to raise the levels of it in the blood.

8. In addition to a diet low in it, this type of regular activity can help lower risk of a heart attack.

9. You can also reduce heart attack risk by not doing this.

10. While it can be found in all animal foods it is never found in any of these foods.

What is this substance that is needed by the body to form hormones, cell membranes, and other body substances? It does not have to be eaten because the body can manufacture all it needs.

It is _ _ _ _ _ _ _ _ _ _ _ .

Make a list of foods that are high in it and a list of foods that do not contain it.

6. Limiting Total Fat, Saturated Fats, and Cholesterol

In the diet, it's the total amount of fat and cholesterol that matters. MODERATION is the key. Don't eliminate all fats completely, but balance high-fat foods with others that contain less fat and cholesterol.

Directions: Below, on the left, is a list of high-fat foods. On the next page is a list of foods lower in fat. Match a lower-fat food with a high-fat food it might replace in a meal or recipe. After completing the match-ups, calculate the calories from fat in the high-fat food and in its substitute. One gram of fat equals 9 calories, so multiply the number of grams of fat in a food times 9. See first item for an example.

High-fat Food	Serving Size	Grams of Fat	Calories from Fat	Substitute Food	Serving Size	Grams of Fat	Calories from Fat
Whole milk	1 cup	8	72	Skim milk	1 cup	1	9
Cottage cheese 4%	1 cup	9					
Ice cream	1 cup	7					
Potatoes au gratin	½ cup	19					
Chicken with skin	3 oz	12					
Buttered snap beans	½ cup	4					
Salad dressing	1 tbsp	9					
Whole milk yogurt	8 oz	7					
Lean and fat roast beef	3 oz	16					
Lean and fat pork chop	3 oz	20					
Tuna salad	1 cup	19					
Bacon	3 slices	9					
Cream of chicken soup	1 cup	7					
Egg	1	6					
Avocado	½ medium	15					
Potato chips	20	14					
Chocolate	1 oz	9					
Sour cream	1 cup	48					
Doughnut	1	13					
Apple pie	1 slice	18					

6. Limiting Total Fat, Saturated Fats, and Cholesterol (continued)

Substitute Foods That Are Lower in Fat

Low-fat Food	Serving Size	Grams of Fat	Low-fat Food	Serving Size	Grams of Fat	Low-fat Food	Serving Size	Grams of Fat
Baked potato	1	trace	Lean only pork chop	3 oz	12	Apple	1	trace
Bacon bits	1 oz	1.3	Banana	1 med	trace	English muffin	1	1
Skim milk	1 cup	1	Air-popped popcorn	1 cup	trace	Low-calorie dressing	1 tbsp	trace
Canned snap beans	½ cup	trace	Egg whites	2	trace	Ice milk	1 cup	3
Chicken without skin	3 oz	6	Chicken bouillon	1 pkt	1	Gumdrops	1 oz	trace
Water-packed tuna	3 oz	1	Low-fat yogurt	8 oz	4	Butter-milk	1 cup	2
Lean beef	3 oz	6	Cottage cheese 1%	1 cup	2			

Name _____ Date _____

7. Complex vs. Simple Carbohydrates

There are nutritionally sound reasons that nutrition guidelines suggest that 50% of our calories come from carbohydrates. Athletes, on training diets, may want to obtain an even larger percentage of their calories from this nutrient.

What are carbohydrates and where are they?

Digestible carbohydrates come from three sources. These are:

1. **Simple sugar alone** (Found in ordinary table sugar, syrups, jellies, etc.)
2. **Simple sugar in nutritious food** (Found in dairy products and fruit)
3. **Complex carbohydrates** (Found in starchy fruits and vegetables and in bread and cereals)

Part I

Below is a list of foods that are rich in carbohydrates.

Directions: To the left of each food, mark what category of carbohydrate it represents (1, 2, or 3).

Form of Carbohydrate	Food Name	Serving Size	Calories	Grams of Carbohydrate	Percentage of U. S. RDA							
					Protein	Vitamin A	Vitamin C	Thiamin	Riboflavin	Niacin	Calcium	Iron
1. _____	Skim milk	1 cup	90	12	20		4	6	25		30	
2. _____	Orange	1	60	15	6	110	8	2	2	6	2	
3. _____	Peas, green	1 cup	110	21	15	60	30	10	20	4	15	
4. _____	Bread, enriched	1 slice	60	12	4			6	4	4	2	8
5. _____	Pizza	1 slice	150	20	15	8	8	2	8	4	15	4
6. _____	Cola	8 oz	90	23								
7. _____	Fruit salad	1 cup	185	48	2	25	8	2	4	8	2	4
8. _____	Potato, baked	1	150	34	6		50	10	4	15	2	6
9. _____	Sugar	1 tbsp	40	10								
10. _____	Gelatin dessert	1 cup	140	34	6							
11. _____	Corn flakes	1 oz	110	24	4	20	20	25	25	20		20
12. _____	Jelly	1 tbsp	50	13			2					2

7. Complex vs. Simple Carbohydrates (continued)

Part II

Directions: Choose one food from each category indicated below and make a bar graph showing the nutrients in that food.

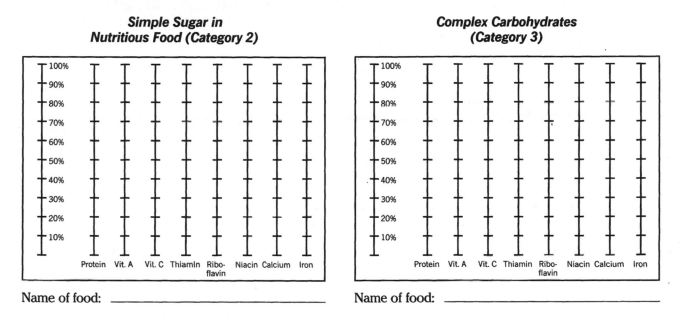

**Simple Sugar in
Nutritious Food (Category 2)**

**Complex Carbohydrates
(Category 3)**

Name of food: _____   Name of food: _____

Part III

How would a graph for a simple sugar compare to the foods you graphed? What recommendation would you make regarding the best way to get the carbohydrates we need in our diet?

8. Eating Enough Carbohydrates

More than one half of our total calories should come from carbohydrates. For an average diet of 2000 calories, that means more than 1000 calories should come from carbohydrates. At 4 calories per gram, that translates into at least 250 grams of carbohydrates a day.

Directions: From the list of foods below, check off enough carbohydrates to give you a day's worth of this nutrient (250 grams of carbohydrates). The number following each food indicates grams of carbohydrates.

Dairy Foods

_____ ½ cup cottage cheese (3)

_____ ¾ cup cocoa (19)

_____ ½ cup ice cream (16)

_____ 1 cup milk (11)

_____ 1 cup chocolate milk (26)

_____ 10.6 oz chocolate milk shake (63)

_____ ½ cup pudding (25)

_____ 8 oz yogurt (16)

Fruits and Vegetables

_____ 1 apple (20)

_____ ½ cup applesauce (30)

_____ medium banana (26)

_____ potato, baked (30)

_____ ½ cup corn (16)

_____ ¼ cup raisins (30)

_____ ½ grapefruit (13)

_____ 1 orange (16)

Breads and Cereals

_____ 1 bagel (28)

_____ 1 biscuit (13)

_____ 1 slice bread, white (12)

_____ 1 piece cornbread (30)

_____ ¾ cup cornflakes (16)

_____ ½ cup noodles (19)

_____ 1 cup pasta (35)

_____ ½ cup rice (25)

_____ 1 hot dog roll (21)

Meat Group

_____ ½ cup beans, refried (26)

_____ 1 cup pork and beans (30)

_____ 1 cup chili (31)

_____ 2 tbsp peanut butter (10)

_____ ½ cup dried peas (11)

_____ 1 cheeseburger (28)

_____ 1 slice pizza (39)

_____ 1 taco (15)

Sweets, Fats, and Alcohol

_____ 1 oz milk chocolate (16)

_____ 1½ cup beer (14)

_____ 1 piece cake, chocolate (40)

_____ 2 tbsp syrup, chocolate (24)

_____ 1 cake doughnut (17)

_____ ½ cup gelatin dessert (17)

_____ 1 tbsp jelly (13)

_____ 1 tbsp honey (17)

_____ 1 slice apple pie (60)

_____ 1 danish pastry (30)

_____ ½ cup sherbet (29)

_____ 12-oz cola (41)

_____ 1 sugar cookie (14)

_____ 8 oz sweet iced tea (22)

_____ 1 tbsp sugar (12)

Where do your carbohydrates come from?

Carbohydrates, from any of the Basic Four food groups, come with lots of other nutrients and fiber. Simple carbohydrates from the fats, sugars, and alcohol group are usually found alone, or with few other nutrients.

1. How many grams of carbohydrate did you have from the fats, sugar, and alcohol group?

2. How many grams of carbohydrate did you have from the other four groups?

Nutrition and Fitness

9. What's in a Name?

**That which we call a sugar
by any other name would be as sweet.**

Sugar can be found in many foods. Sometimes it is listed by other names but it is still sugar. The letters -ose at the end of an ingredient's name, often denote a sugar. Some of the names of sugars that are found listed on labels are sucrose, glucrose, dextrose, fructose, maltose, and lactose. Other names for sugars are honey, corn syrup, high-fructose corn syrup, molasses, and brown sugar.

Directions: In the problems below, the number of sugars to be located is in brackets after the question number. Sugar is an example of a simple carbohydrate. The grams of carbohydrate in each food are listed, as well as the total number of calories in one serving of the food.

   A. Circle the sugars mentioned in each ingredients list.

   B. At 4 calories per gram, calculate how many calories are from the carbohydrate in the food.

   C. Try to guess what the product is. Products include cherry cola, gum, Apple Jacks® cereal, chocolate chip cookies, a cough drop, and gelatin dessert.

1. A. [6]**INGREDIENTS:** flour, sweet chocolate drops, vegetable shortening, high-fructose corn syrup, sugar, brown sugar, dextrose, lactose, modified food starch, skim milk, baking soda, salt, molasses, eggs, flavor, coloring

   B. Calories/serving   180
      Carbohydrate   28g
      Calories from
      carbohydrate   _____

   C. Guess what it is.

   _____

2. A. [3]**INGREDIENTS:** Sugar, gum base, corn syrup, dextrose, softeners, natural and artificial flavors

   B. Calories/serving   10
      Carbohydrate   2.5
      Calories from
      carbohydrate   _____

   C. Guess what it is.

   _____

3. A. [3]**INGREDIENTS:** sugar, glucose, honey, menthol, oil of eucalyptus, lemon oil, tumeric

   B. Calories/serving   16
      Carbohydrate   4g
      Calories from
      carbohydrate   _____

   C. Guess what it is.

   _____

4. A. [2]**INGREDIENTS:** dextrose, sugar, gelatin, sodium citrate, fumaric acid, tricalcium phosphate, artificial color and flavor

   B. Calories/serving   70
      Carbohydrate   17g
      Calories from
      carbohydrate   _____

   C. Guess what it is.

   _____

5. A. [2]**INGREDIENTS:** sugar, oat flour, salt, corn cereal, dried apples, corn syrup, cinnamon, vegetable oil, sodium ascorbate, artificial color, ascorbic acid, BHT

   B. Calories/serving   70
      Carbohydrate   16g
      Calories from
      carbohydrate   _____

   C. Guess what it is.

   _____

6. A. [2]**INGREDIENTS:** carbonated water, high-fructose corn syrup, sucrose, caramel color, phosphoric acid, natural flavors, caffeine

   B. Calories/serving   96
      Carbohydrate   24g
      Calories from
      carbohydrate   _____

   C. Guess what it is.

   _____

10. Carbohydrate Loading

Directions: Read the information about carbohydrate loading. Then answer the questions that follow the information.

The American Dietetic Association recognizes that a high carbohydrate intake prior to competition can be beneficial to some athletes engaging in *endurance* events.

It is generally agreed that the availability of muscle glycogen (a complex carbohydrate) is the limiting factor in endurance competition. When the muscle glycogen is gone, the athlete can no longer perform. In carbohydrate loading, or glycogen loading, high-carbohydrate diets are used to build up a reserve of muscle glycogen. A reserve of liver glycogen is also necessary to reduce the likelihood of hypoglycemia.

When muscles first lose glycogen and then regain it through a high-carbohydrate diet, the glycogen content of muscle is about twice that gained from a normal mixed diet. An athlete's endurance time corresponds to the glycogen content of the muscle. Carbohydrate loading consists of these steps:

a. Depleting the muscle glycogen one week before the event by exercising to exhaustion, using the same type of activity that will occur in the competition (for example, a long-distance runner might run 10–15 miles at maximum speed)

b. Eating a high-protein, high-fat, low-carbohydrate (100 g) diet for three days. Some recommend no carbohydrate during this period, but that can lead to ketosis, an undesirably high concentration of ketones in the blood and urine. Ketones are the product of the breakdown of fat when carbohydrates are not available. The small amount of carbohydrate recommended during the depletion phase is necessary to prevent this effect.

c. Eating a moderate-protein, low-fat, high-carbohydrate (250 g to 525 g) diet for three days immediately preceding the event. During this final step, complex carbohydrates such as pasta, bread, and starchy vegetables are best since they are more gradually absorbed. Large amounts of sugar, candy, soft drinks, and honey are not needed.

Carbohydrate loading must not be used indiscriminately. *It is of no advantage to the athlete in short-time, high-intensity competition.* Because water is held with the glycogen that is stored, the weight gain may be as much as 2.5 to 3.5 kilograms (5.5 to 7.7 pounds). This can lead to a feeling of stiffness and heaviness that can hinder the athlete in competition.

Carbohydrate loading should be used very selectively for high school and college athletes, and rarely, if ever, for early adolescent or preadolescent athletes. Some athletes do not tolerate carbohydrate loading very well and should not attempt it for the first time prior to a competition. Probably the full loading sequence should be used no more than two or three times a year.

An athlete with diabetes or hypertriglyceridemia should consult a physician before adopting a carbohydrate-loading program. Occasional health problems have been observed, including chest pains, changes in the electrocardiogram, and myoglobinuria, following persistent glycogen loading. Although these changes are uncommon, athletes should seek medical advice if they encounter symptoms.

What is carbohydrate loading?

1. How is it done?
2. Why do it?
3. Who can benefit and who can't?

4. How often can it be done?
5. What are some of the harmful side effects?

11. Fiber

Fiber is a currently popular nutrition issue. Many claims have been made about it. Too often, claims are made that sound logical but have not been scientifically proven. It is important that we obtain as much accurate information as possible and then make up our minds about popular nutrition claims.

Directions: Here are some current claims and recommendations that have been made concerning fiber in the diet. Refer to the *Fiber Fact* sheet provided by your teacher. List the facts that support or contradict each claim. Then decide if you would follow the recommendation or believe the claim.

Nutrition claims

CLAIM 1: If you don't eat enough fiber, the colon contents become hard and dry and stay in the colon longer. If cancer-causing agents are present, the colon will be exposed to them for longer periods of time, thus increasing the risk of colon cancer.

Facts that support this claim:

Facts that contradict this claim:

Do you believe this claim is true? Why or why not?

CLAIM 2: Eating large amounts of bran will lower the incidence of heart disease, hemorrhoids, diverticulitis, constipation, and appendicitis.

Facts that support this claim:

Facts that contradict this claim:

Would you recommend that everyone should eat large amounts of bran? Why or why not?

CLAIM 3: Populations that eat large amounts of fiber have no colon cancer.

Facts that support this claim:

Facts that contradict this claim:

Do you believe this claim is true? Why or why not?

CLAIM 4: Even if it doesn't help to eat extra fiber, it can't hurt. We should be buying and consuming large quantities of crude fiber, expecially bran.

Facts that support this claim:

Facts that contradict this claim:

Do you believe this claim is true? Why or why not?

Name _____   Date _____

12. A-Mazed Vitamin

Directions: There is just one way through this maze. Going on the correct path you will cross facts that are true about vitamin A. Going the wrong way, you will cross facts that are not true about vitamin A. After you have located the correct path, list the facts in the correct categories below the maze.

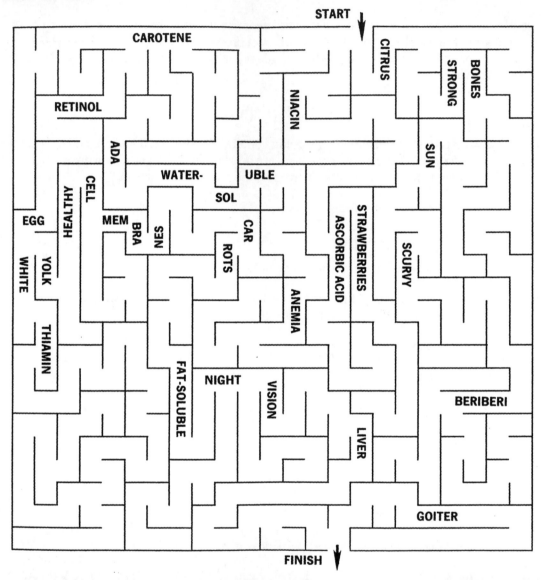

Names for Vitamin A	Functions of Vitamin A	Food Sources	Other Information

13. B Complex

The B vitamins, known as the B complex, have a great deal in common. They also have some individual characteristics.

Directions: Refer to information from your teacher and/or textbook. Record the facts about the B complex, found at the bottom of this worksheet, onto the correct area of this chart.

Vitamin B1   **Vitamin B2**   **Niacin**   **Vitamin B6**

Vitamin B12   **Other B Vitamins**   **True of Most B Vitamins**

Facts about the B complex

1. Also known as riboflavin
2. Also known as thiamin
3. Also known as nicotinic acid, nicotinamide, or niacinamide—never nicotine
4. Also known as pyridoxine, pyridoxal, and pyridoxamine
5. Also known as cobalamin
6. Also known as folic acid or folacin
7. Also known as panothenic acid
8. Biotin
9. Pangamic acid
10. Never bioflavonoids
11. Deficiency causes beriberi
12. Deficiency causes pellagra
13. Used to cure pernicious anemia
14. Found in pork, as well as usual sources of B vitamins
15. Often lost when cooking liquids are discarded
16. It is destroyed by ultraviolet light, so milk, which is a good source of it, should be protected from light.
17. Water-soluble
18. Pregnant women often have a deficiency.
19. Unlike other B vitamins, it is not found in plants, so strict vegetarians can have a deficiency.
20. Needed to release the energy in food
21. Needed for proper metabolic functioning of cells
22. Found in meat (especially liver), whole wheat breads and cereals, milk, and eggs
23. Needed for healthy nervous system

14. Vitamin C

Vitamin C, or ascorbic acid, is needed to promote growth and tissue repair. It helps in healing of wounds. It aids in tooth and bone formation. Lack of this vitamin results in scurvy. Signs of scurvy include lassitude, weakness, bleeding, loss of weight, and irritability. Early signs are bleeding gums and easy bruising.

The RDA for vitamin C is 60 milligrams a day. Extra vitamin C may be needed during stress or pregnancy and if a person has a cold or smokes. Sources of vitamin C include citrus fruits, strawberries, melons, tomatoes, potatoes, and green vegetables.

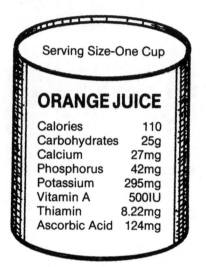

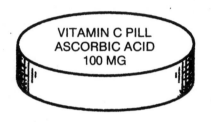

Directions: Use the information above and other sources to answer the following questions on another sheet of paper.

1. Would the pill or the juice provide the most vitamin C?

2. It is possible to obtain pills with very large amounts of vitamin C. When a person has a cold or other infection, is under stress, or smokes, extra vitamin C (but not megadoses of 1 gram or more) may be helpful. Would you advise a person to obtain *extra* vitamin C from a pill or from food? Why?

3. Compare the pill to the orange juice. Which do you think would be the better way to get the vitamin C you need? Why?

4. Your body cannot tell the difference between synthetic and natural ascorbic acid. How does this information conflict with the myth that you should eat only natural organic vitamin supplements?

5. Can extra vitamin C give you pep and energy? Do vitamins contain calories?

6. It is not true that the more vitamins you take the better off you will be. What are the dangers of taking extra-large doses of vitamins?

7. Is it possible to get enough vitamins from food, or is a vitamin supplement usually needed?

8. Vitamin C is water-soluble and is destroyed by heat and exposure to air. How can you avoid losing this vitamin in the foods you eat?

Name _____ Date _____

15. Vitamin E

Of all the vitamins, vitamin E has been claimed to perform the most miraculous feats. Are these claims true or false? Below is a list of facts about vitamin E and a list of claims that have not been proved.

Facts

1. It protects the polyunsaturated fats in the body from destruction by oxygen.

2. It protects vitamin A in the same way.

3. The vitamin is so widespread in food that it is almost impossible to have a deficiency.

4. The body stores great quantities of vitamin E in body fat.

5. Some evidence shows that it provides a measure of protection for animals against lung damage from air pollutants.

6. Vitamin E comes from vegetable oils, wheat germ oil, cereal grains, green plants, egg yolk, milk fat, butter, liver, nuts, and vegetables.

7. Its chemical name is tocopherol.

Many well-designed experiments have been carried out to check the benefits of vitamin E. Following are the results:

8. There is no evidence that it is effective in the treatment of heart problems or muscular distrophy.

9. It does not improve athletic performance.

10. It does not prevent cancer.

11. It does not enhance sexual performance.

12. The oil that vitamin E is dissolved in, not the vitamin itself, may help heal burns and other skin lesions. Also, dermatitis has been linked to the vitamin E in the oil.

13. An increased need for vitamin E is created when extra polyunsaturated fats are eaten. However, the foods containing these fats also contain vitamin E, so extra is not required.

Directions: Each of the claims below has been made for vitamin E. Use the above facts about vitamin E to tell how you could respond to each claim if it were made to you.

Claims

1. Vitamin E cures impotence.
   Your response:

2. A vitamin E deficiency is common and large supplements will be beneficial to your health.
   Your response:

3. Vitamin E protects against heart disease and muscular distrophy.
   Your response:

4. Vitamin E prevents cancer.
   Your response:

5. Using the contents of a vitamin E pill on burns enhances healing.
   Your response:

6. Vitamin E clears skin blemishes.
   Your response:

7. Vitamin E provides the body with energy that it can use during athletic performance.
   Your response:

8. Vitamin E prevents body odor.
   Your response:

16. Potassium

Directions: Unscramble the letters after each item and use them to fill in the blanks beside each question. When you have finished, the letters in the circles will spell the final word of the statement below the questions.

1. Potassium can be lost when an active person exercises strenuously and large amounts of water are lost as _____ .

   N O R I I S P A R E T P

2. A good source of potassium is this citrus fruit juice.

   G R E N A O

3. Because it is high in potassium, this food group may do more for the muscles than meat. It is especially rich in potassium when it is dried.

   I F U T R

4. Potassium is critical to maintaining the heartbeat and in maintaining the body's fluid _____ .

   A C N B L A E

5. Sudden deaths that occur during fasting, in severe diarrhea, and in kwashiorkor (a form of malnutrition) children, are often due to heart failure caused by potassium _____ .

   S O L S

6. These popular starchy vegetables are a good source of potassium.

   A T T S O O P E

7. Loss of potassium in the brain cells, as a result of water loss in the body, is one of the early and most serious consequences of this.

   R A T E D O N I H D Y

8. Except under the direction of a physician, this type of medication (also known as water pills) should not be taken because it causes the body to excrete extra fluids.

   R E S T D U C I I

9. While too little potassium is dangerous, it can be equally serious to have too _____ ; therefore potassium supplements should not be taken.

   C H U M

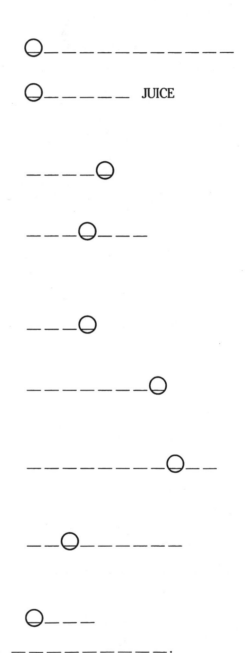

○ _ _ _ _ _ _ _ _ _

○ _ _ _ _ _   JUICE

_ _ _ _○

_ _ _○_ _ _

_ _ _○

_ _ _ _ _ _ _○

_ _ _ _ _ _ _ _○_ _

_ _○_ _ _ _

○_ _ _

A banana is better than a steak when you need _ _ _ _ _ _ _ _ _ _ .

17. Calcium

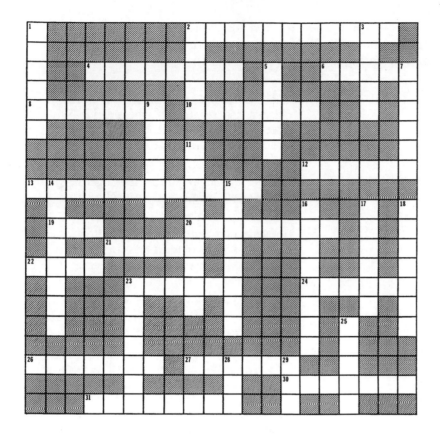

Across Clues

2. These should never take the place of food sources.

4. This nutrient is needed, with calcium and phosphorus, to make strong bones and teeth.

6. This type of soup can be a source of calcium.

8. A disease, caused by a lack of vitamin D, which causes the body to be unable to absorb calcium.

10. This habit can increase the chance of developing osteoporosis.

12. This quick bread is a fair source of calcium.

13. In this disease, bones become thin, brittle, and break easily.

19. For calcium, this is 1200 mg for teens and 800 mg for adults.

20. This, along with a proper diet, is needed for strong bones.

21. Calcium is needed to make these strong.

22. This beverage is an excellent source of calcium.

23. This dairy food is an excellent source of calcium.

24. When eaten raw, these are a fair source of calcium.

26. This popular, natural cooking cheese adds calcium whenever it is used.

27. This substance, which helps hold cells together, needs calcium to be formed.

30. Drinking this beverage increases the chance of developing osteoporosis.

31. This popular process cheese is an excellent source of calcium.

Down Clues

1. This low-calorie substitute for sour cream can be eaten alone.

2. This cheese, with holes, is a good source of calcium.

3. As with bones, calcium is needed to make these strong.

5. All the foods in this food group are excellent sources of calcium.

7. Calcium is needed to make this contract properly. The heart is one of these.

9. If eaten with the bones, this fish can be a fair source of calcium.

11. This type of pasteurized cheese was invented in the USA.

14. If eaten bones and all, these are an excellent source of calcium.

15. This sweet dessert is a good source of calcium and calories.

16. This hormone helps the body absorb calcium.

17. This group of people also needs calcium and dairy products.

18. Calcium is this kind of a nutrient.

23. This soft, unripened cheese can add calcium to a salad.

25. This needs calcium in order to clot.

28. This sex is less likely to develop osteoporosis.

29. When you get this, you also get vitamin D, which is needed so your body can use calcium.

18. Iron

Directions: From the numbered statements, select the best answer for each of the terms related to iron. Put the number in the proper space in the magic square box. The total of the numbers will be the same across each row and down each column. There will be one number that you will not use.

A. Iron-deficiency anemia

B. Pallor

C. Hemoglobin

D. Myoglobin

E. RDA

F. Sports anemia

G. Iron overload

H. Trace mineral

I. Absorption-limiting factors

A	B	C
D	E	F
G	H	I

MAGIC NUMBER = _____

1. Good sources of iron include liver, beef, chicken, fish, some nuts, whole grains, dried beans, egg yolks, tofu, bean sprouts, dried fruit, and broccoli.

2. Lack of healthy color in complexion, inside of lower eye lid, and under the fingernails. It, along with fatigue and headaches, are symptoms of iron-deficiency anemia.

3. Antacids; non-heme iron found in iron-containing foods other than meat; phytates in tea, and in some fruits, vegetables, and whole grains

4. The oxygen-holding protein of muscles. Iron is the crucial element here because of its ability to hold onto or to release oxygen.

5. The state of having more iron in the body than it can handle or needs. Iron can become toxic in this situation. This is why iron supplements should not be taken without medical supervision.

6. 18 mg per day for teenage men and women, and adult women. 10 mg for adult men. The need for iron is higher during periods of rapid growth and it is needed to replenish blood lost during menstruation.

7. The oxygen-carrying protein of the blood. It is found in the red blood cells. Iron is the crucial element here because of its ability to hold onto or to release oxygen.

8. Any hemoglobin concentration below that which is optimal for oxygen delivery in an athlete or very active individual. It is more common in younger male athletes than in adult male athletes. It is more common in high-endurance sports, such as running.

9. A condition caused by the reduction of the size of red blood cells and loss of their color due to iron deficiency

10. An essential mineral nutrient found in the human body, constituting less than .005 percent of the body weight. Iron is one of them.

19. Salt Shaker Game

Salt is 40% sodium. Too much salt gives us too much sodium. Sodium is thought to be related to high blood pressure and risk of heart attacks. The object of this game is to get the lowest possible amount of sodium in the foods you choose.

Directions: In each section below, arrange the foods from the most salty to the least salty. Record your arrangement on the table to the right of the foods. Put the letter of the most salty in #1 and continue until you put the letter of the least salty in #5. When you are finished arranging, get a list of the food's sodium contents from your teacher. Fill in the amount of sodium in food #5. Finally, add all the #5 sodium amounts together. Record your score below the table.

Salt Shake 1
Breads, Cereals, and Grain Products

	Sodium Rank (#1 high)
A. 1 oz corn flakes	1. _____
B. ½ cup cooked cereal, pasta, or rice (cooked without salt)	2. _____
C. 1 slice white bread	3. _____
D. 1 baking powder biscuit (made from refrigerated dough)	4. _____
E. 1 slice apple pie	5. _____ mg

Salt Shake 2
Soups

	Sodium Rank (#1 high)
A. 1 chicken bouillon cube	1. _____
B. 1 cup chicken noodle soup (canned, made with equal part water)	2. _____
C. 1 cup canned chili with beans	3. _____
D. 1 cup chicken and noodles (cooked from home recipe)	4. _____
E. 1 cup Manhattan clam chowder	5. _____ mg

Salt Shake 3
Sandwich Makers

	Sodium Rank (#1 high)
A. 1 oz bologna	1. _____
B. 1 oz ham	2. _____
C. 1 hot dog	3. _____
D. 3 oz fresh meat, poultry, or fin fish	4. _____
E. 1 tbsp peanut butter	5. _____ mg

(continued)

19. Salt Shaker Game (continued)

Salt Shake 4
Fruits and Vegetables

<u>Sodium Rank (#1 high)</u>

A. 1 cup canned green beans (cooked without added salt)　　1. _____
B. 1 cup raw green beans (cooked without added salt)　　2. _____
C. 1 cup frozen green beans (cooked without added salt)　　3. _____
D. 1 cup orange juice　　4. _____
E. 1 cup canned peaches　　5. _____ mg

Salt Shake 5
Milk and Cheese

<u>Sodium Rank (#1 high)</u>

A. 1 cup milk　　1. _____
B. 1 oz American cheese　　2. _____
C. ½ cup cottage cheese (uncreamed)　　3. _____
D. 1 cup yogurt　　4. _____
E. 1 oz cheddar cheese　　5. _____ mg

Salt Shake 6
Snacks

<u>Sodium Rank (#1 high)</u>

A. 20 potato chips　　1. _____
B. 1 cup salted popcorn　　2. _____
C. 10 thin, twisted pretzels　　3. _____
D. 1 dill pickle　　4. _____
E. 10 green olives　　5. _____ mg

Salt Shake 7
Condiments and Seasonings

<u>Sodium Rank (#1 high)</u>

A. 1 tbsp fresh or dried herbs (no salt added)　　1. _____
B. 1 tbsp mayonnaise　　2. _____
C. 1 tbsp mustard　　3. _____
D. 1 tbsp catsup　　4. _____
E. 1 tsp salt　　5. _____ mg

Your total: _____

Rating

909–1099 *Excellent*—You are an expert salt and sodium spotter.

1100–3300 *Average*—This is the recommended range for sodium per day.

3400+ *Poor*—You need to study sources of sodium and salt.

20. Water Test

Directions: All of the true/false statements below are false. On the line under each statement write a correct version of the statement. For example, to make statement 1 correct you could rewrite it as: It is very dangerous to limit water intake before, during, or after strenuous activity.

1. **False:** Going without enough water before, during, and after strenuous exercise does no physical harm.
   True: _____

2. **False:** Water's most important job during exercise is to maintain the body's elevated temperature.
   True: _____

3. **False:** Do not drink cool water every 10–15 minutes before, during, and after exercising.
   True: _____

4. **False:** People who sweat a lot do not need to force themselves to drink fluids. They should rely on thirst to tell how much water to drink and when to drink it.
   True: _____

5. **False:** Drink only undiluted sport drinks that contain sugar, salt, and electrolytes before and during sports events.
   True: _____

6. **False:** Take salt tablets to replace salt lost in sweat.
   True: _____

7. **False:** Wear clothing that prevents evaporation of sweat.
   True: _____

8. **False:** The best time of the day to exercise is from close to noon until mid-afternoon.
   True: _____

9. **False:** Being partially dehydrated does not have any effect on being able to perform at top levels of physical activity.
   True: _____

10. **False:** Dehydration to accomplish weight loss prior to a sports event is acceptable.
    True: _____

11. **False:** Drinking large amounts of water infrequently is better than drinking small amounts frequently (every 10–15 minutes).
    True: _____

12. **False:** Though it makes a person feel clammy, thirsty, and chilled, dehydration does not have long-lasting serious consequences.
    True: _____

13. **False:** Sweating really doesn't cause a person to lose a significant amount of body fluids and thus is not a serious concern.
    True: _____

14. **False:** Having enough fluids before, during, and after sports events is the single most important factor in the success or failure of the athlete.
    True: _____

15. **False:** Warm water is better than cool water. It leaves the stomach faster and helps cool the body.
    True: _____

Nutrition and Fitness

21. Alcohol

Down Clues

1. Containing the stimulant caffeine, this beverage does not help one sober up.
2. This B vitamin is used by the liver to wash alcohol from the system.
3. One and one-half ounces of this equal one drink.
4. Irreversible hardening of liver tissue. One cause is heavy and repeated alcohol use.
5. Drinking alcohol during pregnancy can cause a variety of birth _____ .
7. Also called vitamin B1, it is needed by the liver to wash alcohol from the system.
8. Poor appetite, empty calories in alcohol, and the body's reaction to alcohol can cause this.
13. Limiting amount drunk and sipping instead of gulping are two ways to drink in _____ .
14. The judgment or reasoning area of this organ is the first to feel the effects of alcohol.
18. Those most affected by alcohol are protein, B vitamins, and the minerals magnesium and potassium.
21. The name of the type of alcohol in intoxicating beverages.
23. A highball or a cocktail is sometimes known as a mixed _____ .
26. This is what it takes to sober up. There is no way to speed the process.

Across Clues

4. Every gram of alcohol contains seven of these.
6. Food containing this nutrient is a good thing to eat before drinking alcohol.
9. Alcohol causes a loss of this type of coordination, causing staggering.
10. Three ounces of this sweet wine count as one drink.
11. If you drink, don't do this.
12. When your stomach is full of this, it slows the entry of alcohol into the blood.
15. Alcohol can harm this type of marrow.
16. This is the only organ that can wash alcohol from your system.
17. A feeling of hunger, this is often dulled for a heavy drinker.
19. The center of the brain that controls this is the first to be affected by alcohol.
20. Because of its ability to deaden pain, it was used for years as this.
22. Any drug that dulls the senses, induces sleep, and becomes addictive with continued use.
24. Twelve ounces of this equal one drink. It is not recommended as a beverage for athletes.
25. Not drinking any alcohol ever is called this.
27. An alcohol addict is called this.
28. Five ounces of this equals one drink.

22. Energy

Directions: Unscramble the letters that follow each definition. Place the correct letters in the boxes. The highlighted letters, when unscrambled, will spell the word at the end of the definitions.

1. The amount of heat energy needed to raise the temperature of 1 kilogram (a little over 4 cups) of water 1°C. (This is more accurately preceded by the prefix *kilo*, but is frequently used alone.)

   LIRAOCE □□□□□□□

2. A tool for keeping your weight at the proper point. It is done by keeping the number of calories you eat during a day equal to the number of calories you use during the day. (It is usually preceded by the word *energy*.)

   CLAABEN □□□□□□□

3. Energy needed to carry on basic processes such as building cells, creating energy, and keeping body systems working

   AALBS LAMTOMBISE □□□□□ □□□□□□□□□□

4. The result of eating more calories than the body uses

   THIWGE AING □□□□□□ □□□□

5. The calories found in foods with low nutrient density. These calories provide energy but little else.

   PYMET □□□□□

6. Activities that require the least amount of energy to accomplish

   DEENSYTAR □□□□□□□□□

The key to being able to maintain life, activity, and weight

□□□□□□

Name _____ Date _____

23. Rating Your Diet

DIETARY GUIDELINES FOR AMERICANS
RECOMMENDED BY THE U.S.D.A. & U.S. DEPARTMENT OF HEALTH AND HUMAN SERVICES
Directions: In the chart below list the foods you eat during one day. Use a reference book or a computer to find data about your diet. Total the information.

Food Eaten	Amount	Milk	Meat	Grain	Fruit & Veg.	Calories	Total Fat	Satura-ted Fat	Choles-terol	Carbo-hydrate	Fiber	Sodium
Breakfast												
Lunch												
Evening Meal												
Snacks												
Totals												
Recommended Amounts (where available)		4	2	4	4	2100 (F) 2800 (M)	70 g 93 g		300 mg	305 g (F) 406 g(M)		2000 mg

Consult the information from your diet chart (the specific data to look at is listed in the parentheses) and tell how your diet rates and what you ate that helped you meet or not meet each of the following guidelines.

1. Eat a variety of foods. (Basic Four servings)

2. Maintain ideal weight. (Calories)

3. Avoid too much fat, saturated fat, and cholesterol. (Fat, Saturated Fat, Cholesterol)

4. Eat foods with adequate starch and fiber. (Carbohydrate, Fiber)

5. Avoid too much sugar. (Sources of carbohydrate)

6. Avoid too much sodium. (Sodium)

7. If you drink alcohol, do so in moderation. (Food Eaten, Amount)

24. Balancing with the Basic Four

For a teen, a balanced diet contains:

       4 servings from the milk group
       4 servings from the bread and cereal group
       2 servings from the meat group
       4 servings from the fruits and vegetables group
       A source of vitamins A and C
       No more than 30% of its calories from fat
       Good sources of complex carbohydrate and fiber

Directions: Use the tips above to modify the following day's diets so they balance. You may need to remove and/or add foods.

Big Ben the Body Builder	Missy the Meal Skipper	Dieting Donna	Walt the Wrestler
Breakfast	**Breakfast**	**Breakfast**	**Breakfast**
2 eggs 4 oz steak ½ cup home fries 4 biscuits 8 pats butter 2 cups coffee	No breakfast	1 doughnut 1 cup iced tea	No breakfast
Lunch	**Lunch**	**Lunch**	**Lunch**

2 double burgers, buns,
   dressing
2 cups French fries
1 milk shake
1 apple pie
	1 cup French fries	2 cups salad	1 cup lettuce (no
			   dressing)
			½ cup gelatin

Evening Meal	**Evening Meal**	**Evening Meal**	**Evening Meal**
2 servings meat loaf 1 cup mashed potatoes 1 cup corn ¼ cup gravy 2 glasses milk 2 pieces chocolate cake	1 piece fried chicken ½ cup noodles 1 piece cornbread ½ cup ice cream	2 cups vegetable soup 2 cups cola	2 oz chicken 1 slice bread 2 cups tea with 6 tbsp honey ½ cup gelatin
Snacks	**Snacks**	**Snacks**	**Snacks**
2 candy bars 4 iced teas 2 chocolate milks 2 cups peanuts	2 cupcakes 2 sodas Ice-cream sandwich 2 bags chips	2 sodas 1 dill pickle	No snacks

25. What's an Exchange?

Dietary exchanges are groups of foods that have similar nutrients. Serving sizes are adjusted so calories stay the same. Thus exchanges within a group can be interchanged as desired. Originally designed for use by diabetics, using choices from the exchange groups is now a common way of creating or evaluating diets for all kinds of needs.

The trick is not only to know what foods are in what exchanges (foods are not always grouped the same as they are in the Basic Four groups), but to know how much of each food equals 1 exchange.

Directions: In each exchange below fill in the amount that represents 1 exchange. You will need to refer to exchange lists in your textbook or provided by your teacher.

Milk Exchange

skim/very low-fat
(12 g carbohydrate, 8 g protein, 90 calories)
___ Skim milk
___ Non-fat yogurt
___ Non-fat dry milk powder

Milk Exchange

whole (12 g carbohydrate, 8 g protein, 8 g fat, 150 calories)
___ Whole milk

Starch/Bread Exchange

(15 g carbohydrate, 2 g protein, 80 calories)
___ Bread
___ English muffin
___ Hamburger roll
___ Ready-to-eat, unsweetened cereal
___ Rice (cooked)
___ Yam (sweet potato)
___ Baked potato
___ Graham crackers
___ Popcorn (no fat added)

___ Bagel
___ Plain roll
___ Cooked cereal
___ Grits

___ Pasta (cooked)
___ Corn
___ Pita (6-inch)
___ Pretzels
___ Saltine® crackers

Bread Exchange + 1 Fat Exchange

(125 calories)
___ Pancakes
___ Taco shells

___ French fries
___ Muffin or biscuit

Meat Exchange (lean)

(7 g protein, 3 g fat, 55 calories)
___ Very lean beef
___ Fish
___ Cottage cheese

___ Chicken (without skin)
___ Tuna (in water)
___ Egg whites

Milk Exchange

low-fat
(12 g carbohydrate, 8 g protein, 5 g fat, 120 calories)
___ 2% milk
___ Low-fat yogurt with added milk solids

___ Whole milk yogurt

Meat Exchange + ½ Fat Exchange (medium-fat)

(7 g protein, 5 g fat, 75 calories)
___ Most beef
___ Salmon
___ Mozzarella cheese
___ Tofu

___ Pork
___ Ricotta cheese
___ Whole egg
___ Liver

Meat Exchange + 1 Fat Exchange (high-fat)

(7 g protein, 8 g fat, 100 calories)
___ Pork sausage
___ All regular cheeses
___ Peanut butter

___ Fried fish
___ Lunch meat
___ Frankfurter (chicken or turkey)

Vegetable Exchange

(5 g carbohydrate, 2 g protein, 25 calories)
___ All nonstarchy vegetables (cooked)

___ All nonstarchy vegetables (raw)

Fruit Exchange

(15 g carbohydrate, 60 calories)
___ Apple
___ Banana
___ Grapefruit
___ Mango
___ Raisins

___ Applesauce (unsweetened)
___ Cantaloupe (5-inch)
___ Grapes (small)
___ Orange
___ Orange juice

Fat Exchange

(5 g fat, 45 calories)
___ Margarine
___ Mayonnaise
___ Seeds
___ Olives
___ Coconut
___ Cream cheese

___ Avocado
___ Peanuts
___ Oil
___ Salad dressing
___ Cream (heavy)
___ Sour cream

26. Nutrient Density

The term *nutrient density* means the amount of nutrients a food has in relation to the number of calories it has. All the foods graphed below have approximately the same number of calories, but their nutrient content varies greatly.

Directions: Consider a nutrient-dense food one that either (a) has four nutrient bars higher than the calorie bar, or (b) has two nutrient bars at least twice as high as the calorie bar. An empty-calorie food meets neither of these tests. The calorie bar (1) is a clear bar; the nutrient bars are solid bars. Horizontal lines across the graphs show the height of the calorie bar and twice its height.

1. Use the numbers below the bars to identify the nutrients that (A) are higher than the calorie bar or (B) are at least twice as high as the calorie bar.

2. Decide if the graphed food can pass the test for nutrient density. Circle Nutrient-dense or Empty-calorie.

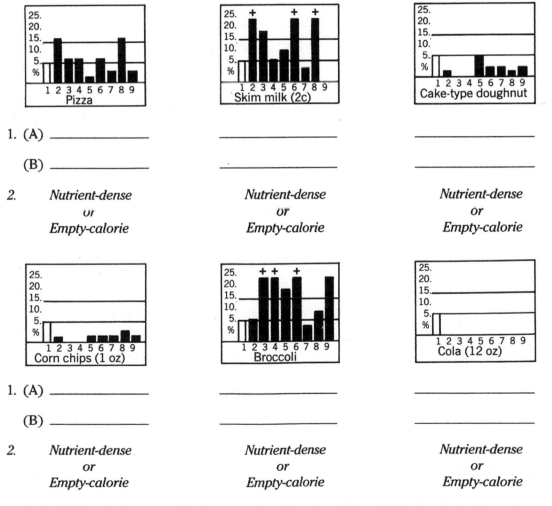

1. (A) _____   _____   _____

   (B) _____   _____   _____

2.   *Nutrient-dense*   *Nutrient-dense*   *Nutrient-dense*
          or   *or*   *or*
     Empty-calorie   *Empty-calorie*   *Empty-calorie*

1. (A) _____   _____   _____

   (B) _____   _____   _____

2.   *Nutrient-dense*   *Nutrient-dense*   *Nutrient-dense*
          or   *or*   *or*
     Empty-calorie   *Empty-calorie*   *Empty-calorie*

Use this information to explain the terms "nutrient density" and "empty calories."

27. Importance of Breakfast

Nutritionists and consumers do not always agree about breakfast. Nutrition experts know that breakfast is an important part of a balanced diet. Many consumers are breakfast skippers.

Directions: Your job is to write a radio or TV ad that will try to convince people they should include breakfast in their daily eating pattern. First, do some consumer research. Survey at least ten friends, family members, or other acquaintances to figure out what may convince breakfast skippers to change. Include the following questions in your survey:

1. How often do you eat breakfast?

    A. Never   D. Almost every day
    B. Seldom   E. Every day
    C. Only on weekends   F. Other _____

2. When you skip breakfast, what is the reason?

    A. No time   D. Nothing available to eat
    B. Makes you feel sick   E. Too many calories
    C. Not hungry   F. Other _____

3. When you eat breakfast, what is the reason?

    A. Have time   E. There's food available.
    B. Hungry   F. It's good for me.
    C. Parent makes me.   G. Other _____
    D. It's made for me.

4. When you eat breakfast, what do you eat?

List answers.

5. What food, if available, would tempt you to eat breakfast?

Directions: After you have done the consumer research, write a radio or TV ad that might tempt the people you surveyed to eat breakfast regularly. If possible, include some menu ideas.

28. Eating Well When Eating Out

_____ 'S PLACE

MENU

_____ _____ _____ _____ _____

_____ _____ _____ _____ _____

_____ _____ _____ _____ _____

_____ _____ _____ _____ _____

SERVING ONLY NUTRITIOUS FOOD

As the owner and chef of your own restaurant,

1. Name your restaurant in the blank space above the menu.

2. Plan a menu in the blanks on the menu. You may include any food that is nutritious. Do not include any empty-calorie foods.

3. Describe at least five things that you as owner and chef could do to ensure that your customers are offered nutritious food.

_____

_____

_____

_____

4. List what you would order from your menu and explain why you would choose these items.

_____ _____

_____ _____

_____ _____

_____ _____

29. The Effect of the Same Meal on Different Individuals

```
┌─────────────────────────────┐
│            MENU             │
│      Quarter Pounder®       │
│   French Fries   Apple Pie  │
│            Cola             │
└─────────────────────────────┘
```

Directions: Refer to the graphs supplied by your teacher (Appendix Sheet VI) to answer the following questions about the nutritional effects of this menu on people with very different needs.

1. Which individual has the most nutrients in excess of 30%? Which nutrients are higher?

2. Which individual has the most nutrients below 30%? Which nutrients are low?

3. Who has the highest percentage of fat and calories?

4. Who is the only one who gets no more than 30% of his or her day's calories?

5. What nutrients are high for everyone?

6. What nutrients are low for everyone?

7. Is this meal nutrient-dense for any of the individuals? (A nutrient-dense meal will have at least four nutrient bars higher than the calorie bar or will have two bars that are at least twice as high as the calorie bar.)

8. What changes in the menu would have made this meal more nutrient-dense?

9. As a result of this comparison, make two general statements that would be true for any individual eating this type of food.

30. Pregame Meals

```
S N A L U X B H E Q N H K O U W J N Z V F
Y N V U H V Z L D O I K V L O M L F J E S
Z X A Y T P M E I V Y O E I P C D N L M O
O V O E X C I T E M E N T L B X K E I C Z
D Y X S D R A N I H Q G Y O I K K L R T S
D T L H F R N R S I H T K J F I K A E Y S
S H T V D E E Q B U X G B S D A L C T R L
G R N Y D F V C W O L Z Z N Y W Z I A T V
V E H O E P E E K G H I E A G S V G W B N
D E R N C Z V A Y C Z Y N O N I U O J O G
D I U Q I L E L I K S I D W F S L L N F A
J T E R P T S Q Q A A H I R Q Q F O M J J
O E G G S E X E Y S K B O Q A D I H U B T
U T F A E I L J Q S I D H S S T V C M R C
V Z K S E X M I L H E N I R S P E Y K I E
C L V Z S H I H Q O Q D R E E F B S K L J
V Z G F W Z R H W L H X G X I Y V P O O H
Z V R B U T U K G M D I Y E E Z X S H W W
N U F J O E P E H Z D I I B W B J B W S H
```

Directions: Fill in the blanks below with the appropriate word. Then find and circle the word in the word-search puzzle above. Answers can be found horizontally, vertically, and diagonally.

1. A large intake of protein can cause excessive urinary excretion leading to _____ .

2. Complex _____ such as enriched breads and cereals, pasta, fruits, and vegetables are an excellent choice for pregame meals.

3. Eat 2–3 hours before an event to allow for proper _____ of food.

4. The stomach should be _____ at the time of competition.

5. Some athletes experience discomfort when they eat foods that produce _____ or that are highly _____ .

6. Contrary to what many believe, the beverage _____ , especially skimmed, can be a good pregame drink.

7. There is no evidence that _____ foods are better than solid foods before an event.

8. Large amounts of simple _____ are not recommended.

9. Consuming large amounts of honey, candy, and/or soft drinks may cause a surge in the release of _____ , leading to hypoglycemia.

10. Foods high in protein and fat such as _____ , _____ , and _____ foods take a long time to digest and should not be eaten as a pregame meal.

11. The _____ effect of a pregame meal is important, so athletes should eat foods they "think" will help them perform at their best.

12. The rate of stomach emptying can be slowed by emotional _____ .

13. It takes about how long to digest the following nutrients: Fat _____ hours; Protein _____ hours; and Carbohydrate _____ hours.

14. When protein is digested, it gives off organic acids that must be eliminated by the _____ .

15. A pregame meal should provide enough _____ so the athlete enters competition well hydrated.

31. *Vegetarianism*

Vegetarians are people who choose diets that are mostly foods from plant sources. Many vegetarians eat some kinds of animal products. Their choice of certain foods determines their name. Vegetarians must study and follow strict nutritional rules so that their diet is balanced. If a vegetarian diet is followed incorrectly, a dangerous deficiency can occur.

Following are definitions of the types of vegetarians.

Lacto-Vegetarian—Will eat dairy products but excludes animal flesh and all other animal products.

Lacto-Ovo-Vegetarian—Will eat animal products such as diary products and eggs but excludes animal flesh.

Non-Meat Eater—Will eat fish, poultry, and animal products such as milk and eggs. Excludes red meat such as beef, pork, or lamb.

Ovo-Vegetarian—Will eat eggs but excludes animal flesh and all other animal products.

Vegan—Will eat only plant foods. Excludes animal flesh and all other animal products.

Zen Macrobiotic Vegetarian—Goes through stages. At each stage additional foods are excluded from the diet, until in the final stage only brown rice and tea are eaten.

Directions: In each of the following lists, by removing one food you will have foods that one of the above vegetarians would eat. Cross out the food that does not belong. Then label the diet with the name of the vegetarian group that would follow that diet.

Example:

Zen Macrobiotic _____

rice, tea beef

1. _____

   nuts   beans   fruits and vegetables   whole grains   beef

2. _____

   pork   nuts   beans   fruits and vegetables   whole grains   dairy products

3. _____

   eggs   nuts   beans   fruits and vegetables   pork   whole grains   dairy products

4. _____

   chicken   fish   eggs   nuts   beans   fruits and vegetables   whole grains   lamb   dairy products

5. _____

   eggs   nuts   beans   fish   fruits and vegetables   whole grains   dairy products

6. What are some reasons that people might choose to go on vegetarian diets?

32. Counting Calories

Directions: In each set of foods below, circle the food that has the lower number of calories.

1. A. Small steak (3 oz)
   B. 1 large baked potato

2. A. 2 tsp butter
   B. 2 tbsp salad dressing

3. A. Small piece chocolate cake
   B. 1 large banana

4. A. 1 oz mozzarella cheese
   (partly skim)
   B. 1 oz cheddar cheese

5. A. 4 oz roast pork
   B. 4 oz tuna (in water)

6. A. 4 oz tuna
   B. 4 oz fried chicken

7. A. 4 oz fried chicken
   B. 4 oz rice and beans

8. A. 1 cup puffed wheat
   B. 1 cup cooked oatmeal

9. A. 1 cup sugar-coated corn flakes
   B. 1 cup commercial granola

10. A. 2 scrambled eggs
    B. 4 pancakes with butter and syrup

11. A. 20 French fries
    B. 1 medium potato with 2 tsp butter

12. A. 1 medium fresh peach
    B. ½ canned peach in heavy syrup

13. A. 1 oz cream cheese
    B. 1 tbsp jelly

14. A. ¼ of a whole cantaloupe
    B. ½ cup fruit cocktail in syrup

15. A. 1 piece carrot cake with frosting
    B. 1 piece angel food cake with ¼ cup
    strawberries

16. A. Regular cheeseburger with roll
    B. ¼ lb hamburger with roll

17. A. Hot fudge sundae
    B. Apple pie (fried)

18. A. 1 cup chocolate milk
    B. 10-oz vanilla milk shake

19. A. 1 cup cole slaw
    B. 1 medium dill pickle

20. A. 5 nachos
    B. ½ cup guacamole

21. A. Beef burrito
    B. Beef taco

22. A. Bread stick
    B. 1 slice garlic bread

23. A. Cheese danish
    B. Bran muffin (bakery-made)

24. A. 1 slice Canadian bacon
    B. 4 slices crisp bacon

25. A. 1 tbsp non-dairy coffee creamer
    B. 1 tbsp non-fat dry milk powder

26. A. 1 piece pound cake ($^1/_{10}$ cake)
    B. 1 piece pineapple cheese cake
    ($^1/_{12}$ cake)

27. A. 4 cups popcorn
    B. 10 potato chips

28. A. 6 oz orange juice
    B. 12-oz cola

29. A. 1 medium apple with peel
    B. ½ cup mushrooms

30. A. 1 slice whole wheat bread
    B. 1 large banana

Name _____   Date _____

33. Energy Balance: The Secret to Weight Control

In the human body calories are needed for:

1. Basal metabolism   2. Digestion of food   3. Energy for activities

Of the three it is easiest to change number 3, the calories needed for activities. Therefore, the amount of activity a person engages in is a critical part of that person's weight control.

Directions: The chart below lists activities and the amount of calories that would be used in 10 minutes doing each activity. Calories are figured for a person weighing 120 pounds or 150 pounds. For example, if a 120-pound person did aerobic dancing for 30 minutes that person would use 92 × 3 = 276 calories. For each problem below the chart, plan a strategy that includes activities that could be done to enable the person to meet his or her weight goal.

Approximate Energy Expenditure

Activity	Calories Used/10 min. 120 lb.	150 lb.	Activity	Calories Used/10 min. 120 lb.	150 lb.	Activity	Calories Used/10 min. 120 lb.	150 lb.
Aerobic dancing	92	115	Eating	12	15	Skiing, downhill	50	63
Basketball	53	66	Gardening	28	35	Skiing, cross-country	65	81
Bicycling 6 MPH	35	44	Golf	46	58	Sleeping	8	10
Bicycling 12 MPH	92	115	Hockey	60	70	Soccer	55	68
Bowling	25	30	Housework	32	40	Standing	24	30
Calisthenics	36	45	Jogging 5 MPH	74	42	Swimming	70	87
Car repairs	32	40	Jogging 7.5 MPH	105	132	Talking	16	20
Carpentry	32	40	Motorcycling	28	35	Tennis	60	74
Chopping wood	56	70	Mowing grass	32	40	Walking 3 MPH	34	43
Classwork	12	15	Office work	24	30	Watching TV	8	10
Dancing fast	92	115	Resting	8	10	Weight training	60	74
Dancing slow	28	35	Sailing	30	36	Wrestling practice	110	140
Dressing	24	30	Shoveling snow	60	75	Writing	16	20
Driving	24	30	Skating	41	51	Yard work	28	35

1. **Losing Weight**   Alison weighs 120 pounds which is high for her height and build. She wants to lose 10 pounds before bathing-suit season arrives. She has determined that she can meet her goal by losing 2 pounds per week. That means she needs to work off 1000 calories each day by increasing her activities. What activities could she do?

2. **Maintaining Weight**   Bob has just finished basketball for the year. He now weighs 150 pounds. He does not want to stop eating anything and he does not want to gain weight. He knows he must substitute activities to make up for the 800 calories he used at basketball practice every day during the season. What activities could he do to maintain his weight?

3. **Gaining Weight**   Carl weighs 120 pounds. He wants to put on weight for football. He is already eating as much and as often as he can. He is very active. He plays basketball every evening after school for 2 hours (640 calories), and he jogs to school and home each day—a total of 4 miles (350 calories). He spends 1 hour chopping wood for his family's stoves (336 calories), and he spends another hour a day working on his car or mowing grass (200 calories). Choose activities he could substitute for some of his present ones so he could use 1000 *fewer* calories a day and thus gain 2 pounds per week.

4. **Controlling Weight**   When trying to control weight, why is it essential to combine exercise with a change in caloric intake?

36   *Nutrition and Fitness*

Name _____ Date _____

34. Diet and Exercise

Those extra calories: How long will it take to work them off?

Directions: Draw a line to connect each food on the left to an activity on the right. You can match any food to any activity. Use each activity just one time. Calculate how long it would take to exercise off the calories in the food, using the activity to which you matched it. For example, if you weigh close to 100 pounds and you matched 1. Milk shake (421 calories) to C. Driving (2.0 calories per minute), it would take 210.5 minutes of driving to use up the calories in the milk shake.

(421 calories / 2.0 calories per minute = 210.5 min)

Note: The number of calories used will vary greatly according to how strenuously you do the activity, your sex, your size, and individual differences in how you react to activity. Therefore, the numbers below are estimates.

Food/Calories		Activity	Calories per Minutes Used in Activity 100 lb.	150 lb.	Minutes Needed
1. Milk shake	(421)	A. Watching TV	0.7	1.0	_____
2. 20 Potato chips	(216)	B. Talking	1.3	2.0	_____
3. French fries	(211)	C. Driving	2.0	3.0	_____
4. 12-oz soda	(150)	D. Car repair/housework	2.6	4.0	_____
5. 3 slices pizza	(450)	E. Dancing or calisthenics	3.3	5.0	_____
6. Beef burrito	(466)	F. Bowling	4.3	6.5	_____
7. Taco	(186)	G. Swimming	4.7	7.0	_____
8. 1 chocolate, caramel, peanut candy bar	(350)	G. Running (6 MPH)	8.3	12.5	_____
9. Quarter Pounder® with cheese	(518)	I. Wrestling	8.7	13.0	_____
10. 1 cup ice cream	(255)	J. Walking upstairs	11.3	17.0	_____

When trying to control weight, why is it essential to combine exercise with a change in calorie intake?

Name _____ Date _____

35. How Many Calories Do I Use for Physical Activity?

This exercise will help you make a rough estimate of how many calories you use for your physical activities daily.

Directions: Record all the activities you engage in for a complete 24-hour (1440-minute) day. **You must account for every minute!** After listing the activity, record the minutes spent doing it under the appropriate energy level.

Clock Time	Activity	Minutes Spent at This Activity Level (See chart below)				
		I	II	III	IV	V
A. Number of minutes at each level. (Total each column)						
B. Average number of calories used per minute		1	2	4	6	9
C. Total number of calories used per activity. Multiply A × B						

D. Total calories used.

Now you can estimate the total number of calories used for physical activity for one day. Add all the C column totals together. The sum of C equals the total calories used for physical activity for one day.

Activity Levels

I. Sleeping

II. Very light exercise: sitting, riding, standing

III. Light exercise: slow walking, shopping, housework, golf, fishing

IV. Moderate exercise: walking, dancing, hiking, bicycling, tennis, baseball

V. Heavy exercise: running, football, climbing, weight lifting, boxing, bicycle racing

Name _____ Date _____

36. The Fat Tests

There are many ways to estimate the percentage of fat on your body. Here are some of the less scientific tests. Any one test by itself can be misleading. The way to best test for fatness is to take several tests and average the results.

Directions: First obtain a copy of the charts you will need from your teacher. Then perform each of the tests described below. Finally answer the questions at the bottom of the page.

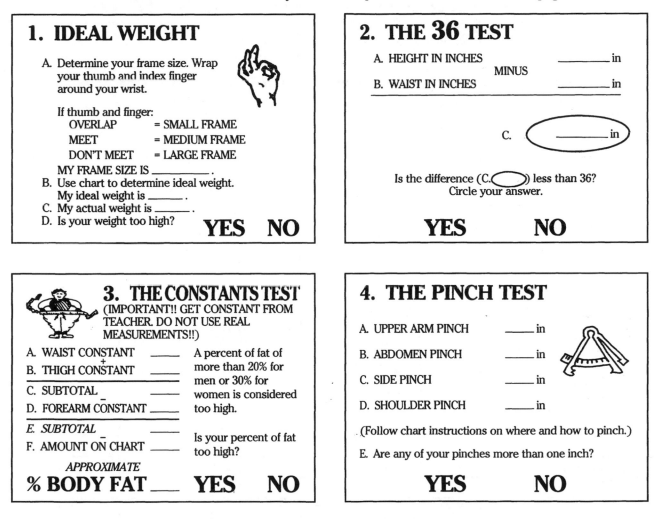

1. IDEAL WEIGHT

A. Determine your frame size. Wrap your thumb and index finger around your wrist.

If thumb and finger:
OVERLAP = SMALL FRAME
MEET = MEDIUM FRAME
DON'T MEET = LARGE FRAME
MY FRAME SIZE IS _____ .
B. Use chart to determine ideal weight. My ideal weight is _____ .
C. My actual weight is _____ .
D. Is your weight too high?   **YES   NO**

2. THE 36 TEST

A. HEIGHT IN INCHES _____ in
                    MINUS
B. WAIST IN INCHES _____ in

C. (_____ in)

Is the difference (C.) less than 36?
Circle your answer.

YES   NO

3. THE CONSTANTS TEST
(IMPORTANT!! GET CONSTANT FROM TEACHER. DO NOT USE REAL MEASUREMENTS!!)

A. WAIST CONSTANT _____
B. THIGH CONSTANT _____
   +
C. SUBTOTAL _____
D. FOREARM CONSTANT _____
   −
E. SUBTOTAL _____
F. AMOUNT ON CHART _____
       APPROXIMATE
% BODY FAT ___   **YES   NO**

A percent of fat of more than 20% for men or 30% for women is considered too high.

Is your percent of fat too high?

4. THE PINCH TEST

A. UPPER ARM PINCH _____ in
B. ABDOMEN PINCH _____ in
C. SIDE PINCH _____ in
D. SHOULDER PINCH _____ in

(Follow chart instructions on where and how to pinch.)

E. Are any of your pinches more than one inch?

YES   NO

Final analysis

The ideal amount of fat for people varies according to age, sex, and activity. Decide if you may be too fat by looking at all four tests. If you answered *yes* to all four tests, you may need to increase activity and decrease calories for a while. (In other words, go on an effective weight loss diet.) If you answered *yes* to just one or two tests, you may just need to do some effective exercises. If you had no *yes* answers, you may be just right or too thin.

As a result of these tests, how would you analyze your body fat?

37. Designing Diets to Lose Weight

Diets to lose weight should be designed so about 2 pounds a week can be lost. This can usually be accomplished for women at 1200–1500 calories a day, for men at 1500–1800 calories. In order to meet nutritional needs, diets to lose weight must supply the same number of servings from the Basic Four food groups that are needed by non-dieting people.

Directions: Choose an amount of calories that would represent a weight-reducing diet for you. Create a day's diet. Use a chart provided by your teacher to determine the number of calories in each food. Make adjustments until your diet has the correct number of calories. Then check if your diet has the correct number of servings from the Basic Four. If it does not, readjust the selection of foods so both the calories and the Basic Four are correct.

Circle your calorie goal.

Female	**1200**	**1300**	**1400**	**1500**
Male	**1500**	**1600**	**1700**	**1800**

Weight-Loss Diet

Food	Amount	Calories	Servings from Food Groups				
			(2) Meat	**(4)** Dairy	**(4)** Bread & Cereal	**(4)** Fruit and Vegetables	Fat and Sugar
Breakfast							
Lunch							
Dinner							
Snacks							
	Totals:						

38. Determining Ideal Weight and Maintaining It

Directions: Refer to an ideal weight chart to determine if the following people need to change their weight. Changes should average 1 to 2 pounds per week. Calculate how long each of them should take to get their weight within the desired range.

Example: Susan, age 14, has a small frame. She is 5′2″ tall. She weighs 129 pounds. According to the chart for girls her age, she should be in the range of 101–109 pounds. She needs to lose 20 pounds. Losing 1–2 pounds each week, it would take her 10–20 weeks to reach her goal.

1. Deanne, age 15, is 5′6″ tall. She has a medium frame. Her weight is 111 pounds. Does she need to gain or lose weight? How long should it take her to get into the desired range?

2. Ed, age 16, is 5′6″ tall. He has a large frame and weighs 150 pounds. Should he plan to lose 20 pounds for wrestling season? How long should he plan to take to lose the weight?

3. Fiona, age 18, is 5′6″ tall. She has a small frame and weighs 143 pounds. Is she above, within, or below the desired range for her? How long should she plan to take to get into the desired range?

4. Calculate your own situation. Are you within the range? If not, how long should it take you to reach your desired weight?

Name _____ Date _____

39. Balanced Diets

Whether you want to gain, lose, or maintain your current weight, your diet can be balanced by the 4–2–4–4 Basic Four plan.

Females need approximately 2100 calories each day to maintain their weight. Males need 2800. In order to lose 1 pound per week, subtract 500 calories each day. To gain 1 pound per week, add 500 calories each day.

Directions: Your job is to add foods to the weight-loss diet below to make it: (a) a weight-maintenance diet (2100 calories female and 2800 calories male), and (b) a weight-gain diet (2600 calories female and 3300 calories male).

Refer to a list of foods and their calorie counts or estimate calories using the exchange system. Use a minimum number of foods that fall into the other category of fats, sugar, and alcohol.

Record your added foods, their calorie count, and the food group to which they belong.

Key to Column Numbers

Calories Added	Dairy	Meat	Fruit and Vegetables	Grain	Fat and Sugar
1	2	3	4	5	6

Female Weight-Loss Diet

BREAKFAST

	1	2	3	4	5	6
½ cup orange juice	56			/		
1 oz enriched cereal	107				/	
1½ cup skim milk	120	/				

DINNER

	1	2	3	4	5	6
1 cup green salad	14			/		
1 tbsp lo-cal dressing	15					/
4 oz broiled fish	205		/			
1 baked potato	132			/		
1 tsp butter	34					/
1 cup skim milk	80	/				

LUNCH

	1	2	3	4	5	6
3 oz hamburger	335		/			
1 roll	120				//	
1 apple	80			/		
1 cup skim milk	80	/				

SNACKS

	1	2	3	4	5	6
1 oz cheese	114	/				
5 whole wheat crackers	57				/	
½ cup popcorn	35					/

Total calories for day <u>1599</u>

Total calories added for weight maintenance _____ (Not to exceed 500)

Total calories added for weight gain _____ (Not to exceed 500)

Total number of added servings from food groups

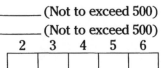

	2	3	4	5	6

39. Balanced Diets (continued)

Key to Column Numbers

Calories Added	Dairy	Meat	Fruit and Vegetables	Grain	Fat and Sugar
1	2	3	4	5	6

Male Weight-Loss Diet

BREAKFAST

	1	2	3	4	5	6
½ cup orange juice	56			/		
1 oz enriched cereal	107				/	
1 cup 2% low-fat milk	218	/				

DINNER

	1	2	3	4	5	6
1 cup green salad	14			/		
1 tbsp salad dressing	65					/
3 oz broiled fish	140		/			
1 baked potato	132			/		
1 tbsp butter	105					/
1 cup low-fat milk	140	/				

LUNCH

	1	2	3	4	5	6
1 double cheeseburger	540	/	//		//	
1 order French fries	251			/		
1 cup low-fat milk	145	/				

SNACKS

	1	2	3	4	5	6
1 oz cheese	114	/				
5 whole wheat crackers	57				/	
½ cup ice cream	145	/				

Total calories for day <u>2301</u>

Total calories added for weight maintenance _____ (Not to exceed 500)

Total calories added for weight gain _____ (Not to exceed 500)

2	3	4	5	6

Total number of added servings from food groups

40. Using Exchanges to Estimate Calories

The dietary exchanges, which were designed to help diabetics plan their diets, can be used by anyone to quickly estimate the number of calories in foods. With a little practice, the exchange system can be a shortcut way to gauge the amount of calories eaten. *Caution:* The exchange system often puts foods in a different group than where they belong in the Basic Four system.

Starch/Bread Exchange
       = 80 calories

Fruit Exchange
       = 60 calories

Meat Exchange
    Lean = 55 calories
    Medium-fat = 75 calories
    High-fat = 100 calories

Milk Exchange
    Skim = 90 calories
    Low-fat = 120 calories
    Whole = 150 calories

Vegetable Exchange
       = 25 calories

Fat Exchange
       = 45 calories

Directions: Use the exchanges to estimate the number of calories each food below would have. Then look up the actual calories and compare your results.

Food	Exchanges	Estimated Calories	Actual Calories
Example 3 oz beefsteak (high-fat)	3 high-fat meat	100 × 3 = 300	330
1. 1 cup whole milk	1 whole milk		
2. 1 small baked potato	1 starch/bread		
3. 1 pat butter	1 fat		
4. ½ cup green beans	1 vegetable		
5. 3 oz broiled chicken (without skin)	3 lean meat		
6. ½ cup broccoli	1 vegetable		
7. 1 hamburger bun	2 starch/bread		
8. 2 tsp mayonnaise salad dressing	1 fat		
9. 1 cup yogurt (low-fat)	1 low-fat milk		
10. 1 small apple	1 fruit		
11. ½ cup cooked rice	1 starch/bread		
12. 2 eggs	2 medium-fat meat		
13. 10 small olives	1 fat		
14. 1 cup skim milk	1 skim milk		
15. ½ white grapefruit	1 fruit		
16. ½ cup grits	1 starch/bread		
17. 10 French fries	1 starch/bread		
18. 1 cup chili with beans	1 fat 1 starch/bread + 2 medium-fat meat + 2 fat		
19. ¼ lb ground beef 21% fat	4 medium-fat meat		
20. ½ cup cooked spaghetti	1 starch/bread		

Nutrition and Fitness

Name _____ Date _____

41. Quick Tricks to Avoid Unwanted Calories

There are some strategies that can help you judge which of two similar foods has fewer calories. By using these as a guide, you will be able to select lower-calorie foods.

Directions: From the list of foods and their calorie counts, choose similar foods, one lower in calories and one higher in calories, that demonstrate each of the guidelines below.

For example, a marshmallow (90) vs. fudge (115) would demonstrate the strategy that light fluffy foods generally have fewer calories than more dense foods.

1. Juice-packed foods are lower in calories than syrup-packed foods.

_____ vs. _____

2. Unsweetened cereals are lower in calories than pre-sweetened cereals.

_____ vs. _____

3. Water-packed meats are lower in calories than oil-packed meats.

_____ vs. _____

4. Broiled or baked meats are lower in calories than meats in sauces or rich gravies.

_____ vs. _____

5. Raw fruits are usually lower in calories than canned ones.

_____ vs. _____

6. Raw or steamed vegetables are lower in calories than creamed ones or ones made with sauces.

_____ vs. _____

7. Thin and watery foods are generally lower in calories than smooth and thick foods.

_____ vs. _____

8. Crisp, non-greasy foods are lower in calories than crisp, greasy foods.

_____ vs. _____

9. Bulky foods are usually lower in calories than compact foods.

_____ vs. _____

10. Nonalcoholic drinks are usually lower in calories than alcoholic drinks.

_____ vs. _____

11. Poultry and fish are usually lower in calories than red meats.

_____ vs. _____

12. Foods cooked in water are usually lower in calories than foods cooked in fat, sauces, or other liquids.

_____ vs. _____

13. Skim milk and foods made with it are lower in calories than foods made with whole milk.

_____ vs. _____

14. Light and airy foods are lower in calories than heavier foods.

_____ vs. _____

Higher-Calorie Foods

Food	Calories
½ cup pears, packed in heavy syrup	98
Chocolate milk shake	355
15 French fries	206
1 piece chocolate cake with frosting	235
1 cup sugared corn flakes	155
½ cup peaches, canned in heavy syrup	100
Bloody Mary with 1½ oz vodka	130
10 potato chips	115
1 chicken pie	545
3½ oz pork chops	360
⅔ cup broccoli with 3 tbsp hollandaise sauce	160
3¼ oz tuna in oil	170
½ cup peanuts	420
½ cup vanilla ice cream	135

Lower-Calorie Foods

Food	Calories
Peach, fresh	65
⅔ cup steamed broccoli	25
Chicken breast, baked	155
1 stalk of celery	5
½ cup vanilla ice milk	93
3¼ oz tuna packed in water	117
½ cup popcorn, lightly buttered	40
3½ oz broiled flounder	70
½ cup pears, packed in juice	60
½ cup tomato juice	25
1 piece angel food cake	135
1 cup corn flakes	95
1 medium potato, boiled	105
1 cup milk	150

Name _____   Date _____

42. A Diet Maze

Directions: Find your way from the beginning to the end of this maze. On your way note the choices and diet tips that lead to success and permanent weight loss. See the example below. Poor diet choices and information lead to dead ends.

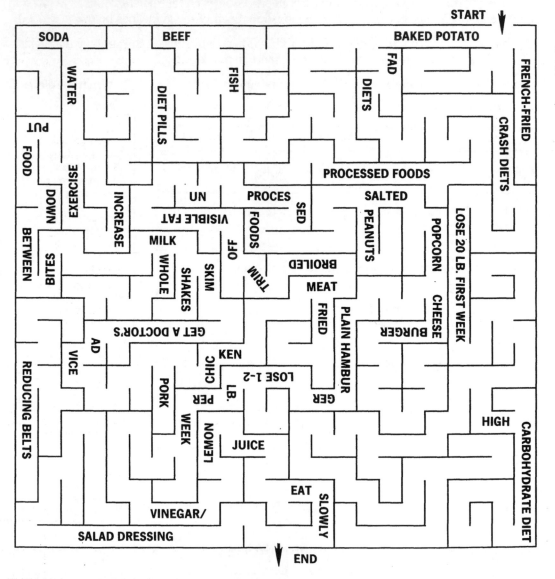

From the maze, list ten good choices to make when dieting.

Example:

1. *Baked potato instead of French-fried potatoes*
    (List nine more on the back of this sheet.)

Also on the back of this sheet, list six good dieting tips.

Name _____   Date _____

43. Fad Diets

It has been said that the only way to lose weight and keep it off is "Eat less and exercise more—forever!" Unfortunately, no matter how much we wish it were true, quick, painless ways to lose weight do not work.

Directions: Each day's menu below represents a popular diet. On the chart at the bottom of the page rate each diet. Record the number of servings provided from the Basic Four. Compare the results to the Basic Four Plan by recording the number of servings the diet is over (+) or under (−) the recommended servings. Use a reference or the exchange system to calculate the total calories for the day. Diet 1 has been completed as an example.

Diet 1	Diet 2	Diet 3	Diet 4
High-Protein Low-Carbohydrate	Quick-Weight-Loss Water-Diet	Grapefruit Diet	Desperate Diet Low-Calorie Repeat same foods.

Diet 1

High-Protein
Low-Carbohydrate

Breakfast
2 eggs
3 oz ham
1 tsp butter
1 cup coffee/cream

Lunch
3 oz shrimp
1 cup green pepper and cucumber
1 tbsp dressing
1 stalk celery
1 oz cheese
1 cup diet soda

Dinner
6 oz broiled steak
1 cup lettuce
1 tbsp dressing
1 tsp butter
1 cup tea/cream

Diet 2

Quick-Weight-Loss
Water-Diet

Breakfast
2 eggs
3 oz hamburger
Coffee

Lunch
1 cup cottage cheese
6 oz chicken
Diet soft drink
8–10 glasses of water per day

Dinner
6 oz boiled shrimp
2 tbsp ketchup sauce
6 oz steak
Tea

Diet 3

Grapefruit Diet

Breakfast
4 oz grapefruit juice
2 eggs
2 slices bacon
Coffee

Lunch
½ grapefruit
6 oz chicken
1 cup lettuce
½ tomato
1 tbsp lo-cal dressing
Coffee
4 oz tomato juice

Dinner
½ grapefruit
6 oz steak
1 cup lettuce
½ cucumber
1 tbsp lo-cal dressing
Tea

Diet 4

Desperate Diet
Low-Calorie
Repeat same foods.

Breakfast
1 cup apple juice
4 oz cottage cheese
2 medium slices melon/lemon wedge

Lunch
1 cup apple juice
4 oz cottage cheese
2 medium slices melon/lemon wedge

Dinner
1 cup apple juice
4 oz cottage cheese
2 medium slices melon/lemon wedge

Basic Four Food Plan	Diet 1 Servings in Diet	Analysis	Diet 2 Servings in Diet	Analysis	Diet 3 Servings in Diet	Analysis	Diet 4 Servings in Diet	Analysis
Milk Group * 4 servings	1	−3(−1)*						
Meat Group 2 servings	5	+3						
Bread and Cereal 4 servings	0	−4						

Fruit & Vegetable
  1 vitamin C source
  1 vitamin A source
  2 or more servings
	1
	0
	3
		=
		−1
		+1						

TOTAL CALORIES	1216							

* For adults (unless pregnant or lactating) use 2.

1. Are any of these diets balanced? If so, which one(s) and why?
2. By just looking at the diets, what can give you a clue that a diet may be a poor choice as an eating plan for losing weight?

44. When Should You Question Nutrition Advertising?

Being a knowledgeable consumer helps you avoid wasting money on products that are of questionable value.

Directions: The numbers in the following ad for Megadol indicate advertising information or techniques that you should question. At each number tell what should be questioned and why.

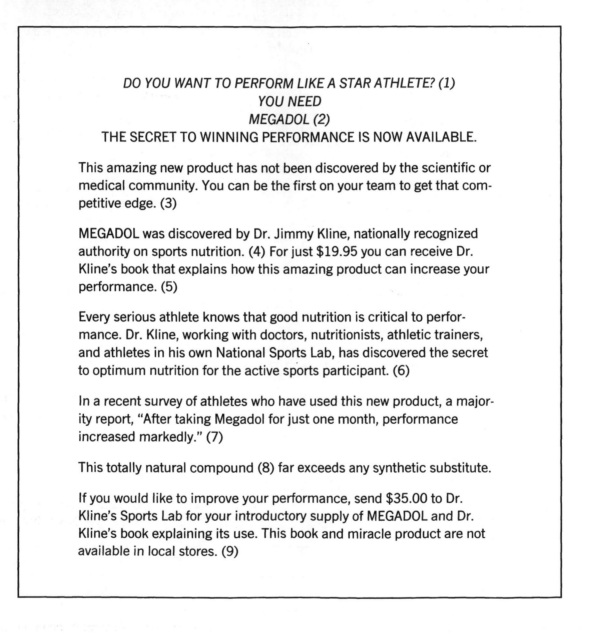

DO YOU WANT TO PERFORM LIKE A STAR ATHLETE? (1)
YOU NEED
MEGADOL (2)
THE SECRET TO WINNING PERFORMANCE IS NOW AVAILABLE.

This amazing new product has not been discovered by the scientific or medical community. You can be the first on your team to get that competitive edge. (3)

MEGADOL was discovered by Dr. Jimmy Kline, nationally recognized authority on sports nutrition. (4) For just $19.95 you can receive Dr. Kline's book that explains how this amazing product can increase your performance. (5)

Every serious athlete knows that good nutrition is critical to performance. Dr. Kline, working with doctors, nutritionists, athletic trainers, and athletes in his own National Sports Lab, has discovered the secret to optimum nutrition for the active sports participant. (6)

In a recent survey of athletes who have used this new product, a majority report, "After taking Megadol for just one month, performance increased markedly." (7)

This totally natural compound (8) far exceeds any synthetic substitute.

If you would like to improve your performance, send $35.00 to Dr. Kline's Sports Lab for your introductory supply of MEGADOL and Dr. Kline's book explaining its use. This book and miracle product are not available in local stores. (9)

45. Nutrient Supplements

Directions: There are widely separated opinions about each topic below. Two extremes of opinion are stated at opposite ends of the line following each topic. Where do you stand on each topic—at one of the extremes or somewhere in the middle?

Place a check mark at the point on the line that shows where your own ideas, beliefs, or opinions fall. After you have marked where you stand on the topic, explain why you positioned yourself at that spot on the line.

1. Taking Nutrient Supplements

I would never take any kind of nutrient supplement. A balanced diet is all that's needed. ——————— Food is not needed. All nutrient needs can be provided with nutrient supplements.

Reason:

2. Nutrients as Ergogenic Aids

Large doses of certain nutrients can improve athletic performance greatly. ——————— Extra nutrients, beyond what the body needs, have no effect at all on athletic performance.

Reason:

3. Importance of Nutrition to Athletes

What an athlete eats is of no importance. Only skill and training make a difference. ——————— The diet of an athlete is the only thing that can make a difference.

Reason:

4. Availability of a Balanced Diet

It is impossible to eat a balanced diet. No one eats such a diet. ——————— A balanced diet is so easy to have that no one needs to be concerned about not having one.

Reason:

5. It Can't Hurt

Nutrient megadoses can't do any damage and they have no bad side effects, so even if they don't help, they can't hurt. ——————— All extra nutrients damage the body and have serious side effects. None should ever be used.

Reason:

6. Sources of Information

The most reliable source of nutrition information is the media. (TV, magazines, commercials, etc.) ——————— The most reliable source of nutrition information is scientific publications.

Reason:

Name _____ Date _____

46. Understanding Nutrition Labels

Nutrition labels are found on many foods. This information can be very useful.

Directions: Refer to the following sample nutrition label found on cereal to learn what information is available and how to use it.

1. What do the initials U.S. RDA stand for?

2. How much cholesterol is in this product?

3. What does the amount of cholesterol present tell about the fat in the food?

4. Can you tell how much sodium is in this product? Why might this be important?

5. Which nutrients are in the cereal but not in the milk?

6. How could you determine if the nutrients were in the cereal ingredients or were added by the manufacturer?

7. What does the ***** at vitamin C mean?

8. How can consumers use this nutrition information?

9. What indigestible carbohydrate is in this product?

10. How many calories come from the carbohydrate in the cereal? (Multiply grams of carbohydrate × 4.)

11. What other nutrition information might be helpful to the consumer?

NUTRITION INFORMATION PER SERVING

Serving size .... 1 ounce (3/4 cup)
Servings per package 14

	1 ounce	1 ounce +½ cup A & D Skim milk
CALORIES	110	150
PROTEIN, g	3	7
CARBOHYDRATE	23	29
FAT, g	1	1
CHOLESTEROL	0	0

PERCENTAGE OF U.S. RECOMMENDED DAILY ALLOWANCES (U.S. RDA)

PROTEIN	4	15
VITAMIN A	25	30
VITAMIN C	*	*
THIAMIN	20	20
RIBOFLAVIN	25	35
NIACIN	25	25
CALCIUM	10	20
IRON	25	25
VITAMIN D	2	15
VITAMIN E	25	25
VITAMIN B$_6$	20	20
FOLIC ACID	25	25
VITAMIN B$_{12}$	25	35
PHOSPHORUS	10	20

* CONTAINS LESS THAN 2% OF THE U.S. RDA FOR THIS NUTRIENT

CARBOHYDRATE INFORMATION

STARCH AND RELATED CARBOHYDRATES	10g	10g
SUCROSE AND OTHER SUGARS	13g	16g
FIBER	3g	3g

Name _____ Date _____

47. Test of Nutrition Knowledge

Directions: For each statement below, circle *T* for *true* or *F* for *false*. Then rate how sure you are of your answer. Circle 1 if you are very sure you are correct, 2 if you are somewhat sure, or 3 if you are not sure at all.

1 2 3   **T F**   1. The six nutrients are protein, fat, carbohydrate, vitamins, minerals, and water.

1 2 3   **T F**   2. Peanut butter is an example of a complete protein.

1 2 3   **T F**   3. Fats from plant sources do not contain cholesterol, but a few of them are saturated.

1 2 3   **T F**   4. Pasta is an example of a food that is a good source of complex carbohydrates.

1 2 3   **T F**   5. All simple carbohydrates in a product are listed in the ingredients as sugar.

1 2 3   **T F**   6. Fiber is an essential part of a balanced diet.

1 2 3   **T F**   7. The fat-soluble vitamins are vitamin B and vitamin C.

1 2 3   **T F**   8. Most people's diets are deficient enough to require them to take nutrient supplements to be more healthy.

1 2 3   **T F**   9. Two minerals that are frequently lacking in a standard diet are calcium and iron.

1 2 3   **T F**   10. A dill pickle has more salt in it than 20 potato chips.

1 2 3   **T F**   11. An athlete should not drink water during heavy exercise.

1 2 3   **T F**   12. A nutrient-dense food is one which has a lot of nutrients in relation to the number of calories it contains.

1 2 3   **T F**   13. One gram of alcohol provides 9 calories.

1 2 3   **T F**   14. A diet designed for weight loss should not cause a loss of more than 2 pounds per week.

1 2 3   **T F**   15. One vegetable exchange is ½ cup of cooked vegetables and averages 25 calories.

1 2 3   **T F**   16. Fast foods are considered junk foods or empty-calorie foods.

1 2 3   **T F**   17. Effective diets often eliminate at least one food group.

1 2 3   **T F**   18. The Basic Four Plan recommends four servings from the meat group each day.

1 2 3   **T F**   19. Testimonials about nutrient-related products are a reliable source of information.

1 2 3   **T F**   20. Nutrition labels state the number of grams of protein in a serving of the product.

Name _____ Date _____

48. The Nutrients

Directions: Below the six nutrient names there are blanks. Below these are 30 statements, each of which describes a characteristic or fact related to one of the nutrients. Put the number that is to the left of each statement on the blank under the nutrient to which it applies.

Carbohydrate   **Fat**   **Protein**

____ ____ ____   ____ ____   ____ ____

____ ____   ____ ____   ____ ____

Vitamins   **Water**   **Minerals**

____ ____ ____   ____ ____ ____   ____ ____ ____

____ ____   ____ ____   ____ ____

Statements

1. It is needed for growth, repair, and maintenance of body tissues.
2. It is the most critical nutrient for active people.
3. Sodium and potassium can be lost by heavy sweating.
4. Its major role is supplying energy.
5. It is the most concentrated energy source.
6. Increased need for ascorbic acid can easily be met by the diet.
7. It is essential for *all* body processes.
8. Sodium and potassium are examples.
9. These are the best source of additional calories for active people.
10. Excess water-soluble ones are excreted by the body.
11. It carries vitamins A, D, E, and K.
12. It is not true that eating extra amounts of this will increase muscle mass.
13. It is necessary for controlling body temperature.
14. The use of salt tablets is not recommended for replacement of this.
15. Like carbohydrate, it is changed to fat when there is too much for the body to use.
16. Complex ones include breads, pasta, fruit, and vegetables.
17. It is the most slowly digested nutrient.
18. Fat-soluble ones are retained and stored.
19. A gram of this or of protein has the same number of calories.
20. Large quantities of A or D can be toxic and sometimes fatal.
21. This nutrient may need to be limited before strenuous activity.
22. Calcium is an example.
23. If used as a fuel source, it will cause fatigue faster than fat or carbohydrate.
24. If not replaced, it can lead to heat exhaustion.
25. Iron is an example and is often deficient in people's diets.
26. Should be drunk before, during, and after hot-weather exercise.
27. Two servings of meat a day will provide extra _____ .
28. Simple ones include sugar, molasses, honey, and corn syrup.
29. This nutrient should not provide more than 30% of the calories for a day.
30. Dark green and yellow fruits and vegetables are a good source of these.

49. Is It Nutrition Fiction or Nutrition Fact?

Directions: For each statement, circle *T* for *true* or *F* for *false*. Change each false statement so it will be a true statement.

T F 1. Extra protein in the diet is used to build extra muscles.

T F 2. Protein has the same number of calories per gram as carbohydrate (sugar or starch).

T F 3. A peanut butter sandwich served with milk provides protein of the same quality as that found in a steak.

T F 4. Foods that contain no cholesterol are lower in fat and calories than foods that contain cholesterol.

T F 5. Polyunsaturated fat and saturated fat have the same number of calories per gram.

T F 6. Potatoes are fattening.

T F 7. Honey or a candy bar can provide quick energy.

T F 8. Water is the most critical nutrient for athletes and they should drink it before, during, and after exercise.

T F 9. Physical activity increases the need for most vitamins.

T F 10. Megadoses of vitamin E can increase physical performance.

T F 11. A banana is better than a steak when you need potassium.

T F 12. People who exercise frequently need to take salt tablets.

T F 13. The American diet often has too few calories from carbohydrate.

T F 14. An empty-calorie food has no nutrients.

T F 15. The most effective way to lose weight is to burn up more calories than you take in.

T F 16. It is possible for a person to lose five pounds of fat during a strenuous workout.

T F 17. Fiber content should be considered when planning a daily diet.

T F 18. Steak and eggs would be a good breakfast before participating in an athletic event.

T F 19. Skipping breakfast is a good way to cut calories, thus helping a person lose weight.

T F 20. The best diet for all people is a balanced diet supplied from a variety of foods.

50. Nutrition Attitudes

Directions: There are widely separated opinions about each topic below. Extremes of opinion are stated at opposite ends of the line following each topic. Where do you stand on each topic—at one of the extremes or somewhere in the middle? Place a check mark at the point on the line that shows where your own ideas, beliefs, or opinions fall. After you have marked where you stand on the topic, circle the word that best describes what has influenced you to position yourself at that spot on the line.

1. Importance of Nutrition

I think how I choose the foods I eat has a great effect on how I feel and perform.

_____

Nutrition does not have anything to do with how I feel or perform.

Family   School   Media   Friends   Personal experience   Other _____

2. Food Preferences

I like almost every kind of food.

_____

I am very fussy. There are a lot of foods I don't like.

Family   School   Media   Friends   Personal experience   Other _____

3. Opinion About New Foods

I enjoy trying new foods.

_____

I do not try unfamiliar foods.

Family   School   Media   Friends   Personal experience   Other _____

4. Eating for Good Nutrition

I try to eat what I know is good for me.

_____

I only eat what I like. It doesn't matter if it is not good for me.

Family   School   Media   Friends   Personal experience   Other _____

Name _____ Date _____

50. Nutrition Attitudes (continued)

5. Interest in Nutrition

I am very interested in
learning about all facets
of nutrition.

I think studying nutrition
is boring.

Family   School   Media   Friends   Personal experience   Other _____

6. Information Reliability

I feel I know when nutri-
tion information is reliable. I am selective about
what I believe about
nutrition.

I never know who to
believe about nutrition. I
usually believe anything I
hear.

Family   School   Media   Friends   Personal experience   Other _____

7. Nutrition Knowledge

I feel I am very knowl-
edgeable about nutrition.

I do not know much about
nutrition.

Family   School   Media   Friends   Personal experience   Other _____

8. Who Has the Most Influence on Your Attitudes About Nutrition?

Look over how you answered the questions above. How have your attitudes about nutrition
developed? Who has the greatest effect on your attitudes?

Appendix I. Fiber Facts

(To be used with worksheet 11.)

1. Fiber is a complex carbohydrate. The links between the sugar molecules in dietary fiber cannot be broken by the human digestive system. Thus, fiber passes down the intestinal tract and forms bulk for the stool.

2. Dietary fiber is the part of plants that humans can't digest.

3. Fiber helps the digestive system work properly.

4. There are several types of fiber, such as cellulose, pectin, lignin, and gums. Plants differ in the types and amounts of fiber they contain.

5. Different types of fiber function differently in the body. It is important to eat a variety of plant foods to benefit from the effects of different kinds of fiber.

6. Bran (wheat fiber) experiments have shown that bran does not have the same positive effects as do other types of fiber.

7. Some types of fiber have a laxative effect, producing softer, bulkier stools and more rapid movement of wastes through the intestine.

8. Fiber is helpful in preventing and treating constipation and diverticular disease.

9. The possible benefits of dietary fiber for colon cancer, heart disease, diabetes, and obesity are being studied. Whether such benefits exist is not yet known.

10. It is not clear exactly how much and what types of fiber we need in our diets daily. However, for most Americans, a moderate increase in dietary fiber by eating more fiber-containing foods like those listed on this page is desirable.

11. There is no reason to take fiber supplements or to add fiber to foods that do not already contain it.

12. Following are some foods high in fiber: whole grain breads and cereals, whole wheat pasta, vegetables (especially with edible skins), stems or seeds, dried beans and peas, whole fruits (especially with edible skins or seeds), and nuts and seeds.

13. Foods high in fiber are not necessarily coarse in texture. Japanese miso (bean paste) and tofu (bean curd) are smooth and soft but very high in fiber.

14. Adding extra fiber (12 to 28 grams per day), especially in purified form (bran) to the diet, is not advised. However, there appears to be little risk in shifting toward the use of more foods that are naturally high in fiber, thus increasing our current 4 grams per day to 5 or 6 grams per day.

15. Appendicitis has decreased in the U.S. as fiber has disappeared from the diet.

16. A low-fiber diet means a high-fat and high-protein diet. Perhaps high fat and high protein are what correlates with cancer.

17. Chromium and zinc disappear when cereals are refined. Perhaps this is the causative factor in the ratio of low-fiber diet to disease.

18. Fiber is the food constituent that reaches the colon.

19. Africans with a high-fiber diet do not have colon diseases.

20. People in India who have a higher-fiber diet also have a higher rate of colon cancer.

21. Constipated people do not have more colon cancer.

22. Studies suggest that a large amount of fiber may have ill effects. It can aggravate, rather than help, constipation due to spastic colon. It can also produce a deficiency of trace elements.

Nutrition and Fitness

Appendix II. Sources of Iron

(To be used for additional information related to worksheet 18.)

Sources of Iron

Food	Serving Size	Iron (mg)
Meat Group		
Meat		
1. Oysters	¾ cup	10.00
2. Beef liver	3 oz	8.00
3. Hamburger	3 oz	2.70
4. Ham	3 oz	2.20
5. Tuna	3 oz	1.00
6. Lamb	3 oz	1.40
7. Chicken	3.5 oz	1.04
Meat Substitutes		
8. Dried beans	½ cup	2.50
9. Tofu	4 oz	2.30
10. White beans (cooked)	½ cup	1.50
11. Egg	1	1.10
12. Filberts	1 oz	0.90
13. Peanut butter	2 tbsp	0.60
Bread and Cereal Group		
14. Bran flakes (enriched)	½ cup	6.20
15. Rice	½ cup	0.90
16. Whole wheat bread	1 slice	0.80
17. Spaghetti, enriched	1 cup	0.70
18. Macaroni	1 cup	0.70
Fruits and Vegetables Group		
19. Prune juice	¼ cup	2.60
20. Spinach	½ cup	2.40
21. Lima beans	3 oz	2.20
22. Mustard greens	½ cup	1.30
23. Dried apricots	4 halves	0.80
24. Broccoli	½ cup	0.70
25. Bean sprouts	½ cup	0.45

Note: The dairy group is lacking in iron.

Appendix III. Salt Shaker Game Answer Sheet

(To be used with worksheet 19.)

Foods are listed from one with largest amount of sodium to one with least sodium last. Milligrams of sodium are in brackets.

Salt Shake 1
Breads, Cereals, and Grain Products

E. 1 slice apple pie [476 mg]
A. 1 oz corn flakes [351 mg]
D. 1 baking powder biscuit (made from refrigerated dough) [249 mg]
C. 1 slice white bread [129 mg]
B. ½ cup cooked cereal, pasta, or rice (cooked without salt) [5 mg]

Salt Shake 2
Soups

E. 1 cup Manhattan clam chowder [1808 mg]
C. 1 cup canned chili with beans [1354 mg]
B. 1 cup chicken noodle soup (canned, made with equal part water) [1106 mg]
A. 1 chicken bouillon cube [960 mg]
D. 1 cup chicken and noodles (cooked from home recipe) [600 mg]

Salt Shake 3
Sandwich Makers

B. 3 oz ham [1009 mg]
C. 1 hot dog [504 mg]
A. 1 oz bologna [360 mg]
E. 1 tbsp peanut butter [100 mg]
D. 3 oz fresh meat, poultry, or fin fish [90 mg]

Salt Shake 4
Fruits and Vegetables

A. 1 cup canned green beans (cooked without added salt) [339 mg]
C. 1 cup frozen green beans (cooked without added salt) [18 mg]
E. 1 cup canned peaches [15 mg]
B. 1 cup raw green beans (cooked without added salt) [4 mg]
D. 1 cup orange juice [2 mg]

Salt Shake 5
Milk and Cheese

C. ½ cup cottage cheese, uncreamed [450 mg]
B. 1 oz American cheese [406 mg]
E. 1 oz cheddar cheese [176 mg]
D. 1 cup yogurt [133 mg]
A. 1 cup milk [120 mg]

Salt Shake 6
Snacks

D. 1 dill pickle [1930 mg]
C. 10 thin, twisted pretzels [966 mg]
E. 10 green olives [950 mg]
A. 20 potato chips [400 mg]
B. 1 cup salted popcorn [86 mg]

Salt Shake 7
Condiments and Seasonings

E. 1 tsp salt [2350 mg]
C. 1 tbsp mustard [190 mg]
D. 1 tbsp catsup [180 mg]
B. 1 tbsp mayonnaise [90 mg]
A. 1 tbsp fresh or dried herbs, no salt added [6 mg]

BEST POSSIBLE SCORE: 909
WORST POSSIBLE SCORE: 8362

Name _____   Date _____

Appendix IV. The Basic Four

(To be used with worksheets 23, 24, 37, 39, 43.)

Dairy Group

Servings Needed Each Day

Teens — 4
Age 9–12 — 3
Age 0–9 — 2–3
Adult — 2

What's a Serving?

1 cup any kind of milk (8 oz, 1 glass)
1½ cups ice cream or ice milk
1⅓ oz cheddar or Swiss cheese
2 oz processed cheese food (2 slices)
2 cups cottage cheese
1 cup yogurt

Bread and Cereal Group

Servings Needed Each Day

4

What's a Serving?

1 slice bread
1 small roll or biscuit
½ hard roll
½ cup to ¾ cup cooked cereal or pasta
½ hamburger or hot dog roll
1 oz ready-to-eat cereal
1 piece cornbread
5 crackers
1 small muffin
½ cup cooked rice
1 slice pizza crust
1 tortilla
1 medium potato

Meat Group

Servings Needed Each Day

2

What's a Serving?

2–3 oz cooked meat, fish, or poultry
2 eggs
1 cup dried beans or dried peas
4 tbsp peanut butter
1 hamburger patty
½ to 1 cup nuts

Fruits and Vegetables Group

Servings Needed Each Day

4

What's a Serving?

½ cup cooked fruit or vegetable
½ cup juice
1 cup raw fruit or vegetable
1 small apple, orange, pear
¼ melon
½ grapefruit

Name _____ Date _____

Appendix V. The Exchanges

(To be used with worksheets 25, 37, 39, 40, 43.)

Each day teens should consume 4 milk exchanges, 4 bread exchanges, a total of 4 fruit or vegetable exchanges (2 vegetable and 2 fruit), 5 meat exchanges, and not more than 3 fat exchanges.

Skim Milk Exchange
12 g carbohydrate, 8 g protein, 0 g fat (90 calories)
1 cup skim milk
1 cup non-fat yogurt
⅓ cup non-fat dry milk powder

Low-Fat Milk Exchange
12 g carbohydrate, 8 g protein, 5 g fat (120 calories)
1 cup 2% milk
1 cup low-fat yogurt with added nonfat milk solids

Whole Milk Exchange
12 g cabohydrate, 8 g protein, 8 g fat (150 calories)
1 cup whole milk   1 cup whole milk yogurt

Starch/Bread Exchange
15 g carbohydrate, 3 g protein (80 calories)

1 slice bread or 1 small roll	1 small bagel
1 English muffin	1 plain roll
½ hamburger roll	½ cup cooked cereal
¾ cup ready-to-eat, unsweetened cereal	½ cup grits
	½ cup pasta (cooked)
⅓ cup rice (cooked)	½ cup corn
⅓ cup yam (sweet potato)	1 pita (6-inch)
1 small baked potato	¾ oz pretzels
3 graham crackers	6 Saltine® crackers
3 cups popcorn (no fat added)	

Bread Exchange +1 Fat Exchange
(125 calories)

2 pancakes	10 French fries
2 taco shells	1 muffin or biscuit

Lean Meat Exchange
7 g protein, 3 g fat (55 calories)

1 oz very lean beef	1 oz chicken (without skin)
1 oz fish	¼ cup tuna (in water)
¼ cup cottage cheese	3 egg whites

Medium-Fat Meat Exchange
7 g protein, 5 g fat (75 calories)

1 oz most beef	1 oz pork
¼ cup salmon	1 oz ricotta cheese
1 oz mozzarella cheese	1 whole egg
4 oz tofu	1 oz liver

High-Fat Meat Exchange
7 g protein, 8 g fat (100 calories)

1 oz pork sausage	1 oz fried fish
1 oz all regular cheeses	1 oz lunch meat
1 tbsp peanut butter	1 frankfurter (chicken or turkey)

Vegetable Exchange
5 g carbohydrate, 2g protein (25 calories)

½ cup all non-starchy vegetables (cooked)	1 cup all non-starchy vegetables (raw)
½ cup tomatoes or tomato juice	

Fruit Exchange
15 g carbohydrate, (60 calories)

1 apple	⅓ cantaloupe (5-inch) or two med. slices
⅓ cup apple juice	
½ banana	15 grapes (small)
½ grapefruit	1 orange
½ mango	½ cup orange juice
2 tbsp raisins	
½ cup applesauce (unsweetened)	

Fat Exchange
5 g fat (45 calories)

1 tsp margarine or butter	⅛ avocado
1 tsp mayonnaise	20 small peanuts
1 tbsp seeds	1 tsp oil
20 small olives	1 tbsp salad dressing
2 tbsp coconut	1 tbsp cream (heavy)
1 tbsp cream cheese	1 tbsp sour cream
1 strip bacon	

Nutrition and Fitness

Name _____   Date _____

Appendix VI. The Effects of the Same Meal on Different Individuals

(To be used with worksheet 29.)

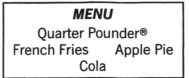

MENU
Quarter Pounder®
French Fries   Apple Pie
Cola

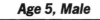

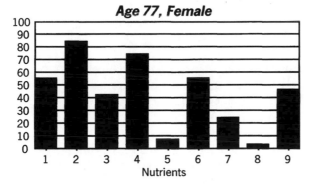

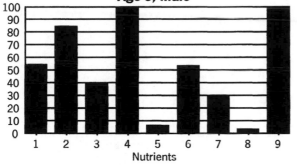

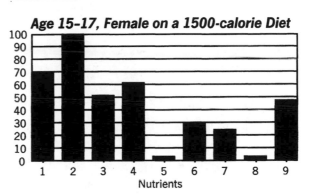

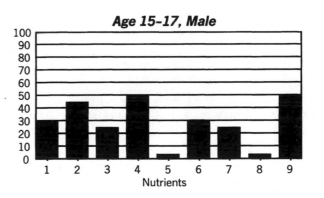

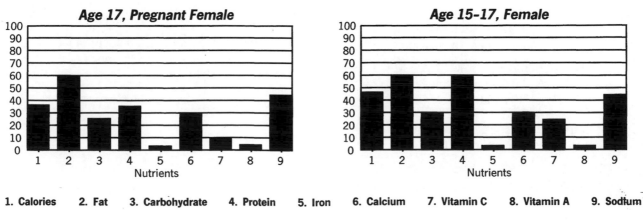

1. Calories   2. Fat   3. Carbohydrate   4. Protein   5. Iron   6. Calcium   7. Vitamin C   8. Vitamin A   9. Sodium

         Nutrition and Fitness

Name _____   Date _____

Appendix VII. Instructions for Using the Fat Tests

(To be used with Worksheet 36.)

TEST 1: Ideal Weight

Refer to an ideal-weight chart (appendix sheet IX). Choose the correct column for your age, sex, and frame size. Choose the row for your height. The intersection will be your ideal weight. Record your ideal and actual weight.

TEST 2: The 36 Test

Just measure your waist and your height in inches. Then subtract your waist measurement from your height measurement. An answer greater than 36 indicates an appropriate amount of fat.

TEST 3: The Constants Test

Refer to the correct constants chart for your sex (appendix sheet VIII). The directions here are lettered to correspond to worksheet 36.

A. Measure your waist ½ inch above your navel. Find the constant that corresponds to your measurement. *Note:* Record the constant—not your measurement!

B. *Girls:* Measure your right thigh just below the buttocks.

Boys: Measure your right upper arm halfway between the shoulder and the elbow, with the arm straight. Find the constant that corresponds to your measurement. *Note:* Record the constant—not your measurement!

D. Measure your right forearm (the widest part between the elbow and the wrist). Find the constant that corresponds to your measurement. *Note:* Record the constant—not your measurement!

F. Amount to subtract:
Girls –20 (Female athletes use –23)
Boys –10 (Male athletes use –14)

Complete the necessary arithmetic to estimate your percentage of fat.

TEST 4: The Pinch Test

Use skinfold calipers if available.

A. With your arm at your side, pinch the skin on the back of upper arm halfway between elbow and shoulder. Do not get muscle in the fold. Carefully remove your thumb and index finger, maintaining the distance between them. Measure between your thumb and index finger. Record measurement.

Repeat this test on your abdomen, near the navel, just over the hip bone at your side, and just over your shoulder blade on your back. Record results.

Ideal percents of fat according to the American Dietetic Association are as follows:
Women: 12% to 25%
Men: 7% to 15%

(Athletes will have lower percentages.)

How much fat is too much? A percent of fat over 30% for women and 20% for men is considered too high.

Appendix VIII. Constants

(To be used with worksheet 36.)

Females 15 to 17 Years Old

Waist		Thigh		Forearm	
Measure Inches	Constant	Measure Inches	Constant	Measure Inches	Constant
20	27	14	29	6	26
21	28	15	31	7	30
22	29	16	33	8	34
23	31	17	35	9	39
24	32	18	37	10	43
25	33	19	40	11	47
26	35	20	42	12	52
27	36	21	44	13	56
28	37	22	46	14	60
29	39	23	48	15	65
30	40	24	50	16	69
31	41	25	52	17	73
32	43	26	54	18	78
33	44	27	56	19	82
34	45	28	58	20	86
35	47	29	60		
36	48	30	62		
37	49	31	65		
38	51	32	67		
39	52	33	69		
40	53	34	71		

Males 15 to 17 Years Old

Waist		Upper Arm		Forearm	
Measure Inches	Constant	Measure Inches	Constant	Measure Inches	Constant
21	28	7	26	7	38
22	29	8	30	8	43
23	31	9	33	9	49
24	33	10	37	10	54
25	34	11	41	11	60
26	35	12	44	12	65
27	37	13	48	13	71
28	38	14	52	14	76
29	39	15	56	15	81
30	40	16	59	16	87
31	41	17	63	17	92
32	42	18	67	18	98
33	43	19	70	19	103
34	45	20	74	20	109
35	46	21	78	21	114
36	47	22	81	22	119
37	49				
38	50				
39	51				
40	52				
41	54				
42	55				

Adapted from National Dairy Council Materials

Name _____   Date _____

Appendix IX. Height and Weight Charts

(To be used with worksheets 36 and 38.)

National Dairy Council's Compilation Based on National Statistics *Height and Weight of Youths 12-17 Years* (1973) and Metropolitan Life Insurance Company's *Desirable Weight*

Height (without shoes)	Weight (with indoor clothing, in pounds) Frame small	medium	large
4'8"	85–91	89–90	97–112
4'9"	87–94	91–103	99–115
4'10"	89–97	94–106	102–118
4'11"	92–100	97–109	105–121
5'0"	95–103	100–112	108–124
5'1"	98–106	103–115	111–127
5'2"	101–109	106–119	114–131
5'3"	104–112	109–123	118–135
5'4"	107–116	113–128	122–139
5'5"	111–120	117–132	126–143
5'6"	115–124	121–136	130–147
5'7"	119–128	125–140	134–151
5'8"	123–133	129–144	138–156
5'9"	127–137	133–148	142–161
5'10"	131–141	137–152	146–166
5'11"	135–145	141–156	150–171
6'0"	139–149	145–160	154–176

Adults
Institute of Human Nutrition/Columbia University *Your Frame Size and Weight* (1955)

Height (without shoes)	Weight (With indoor clothing, in pounds) Frame small	medium	large
Women			
4'10"	102–111	109–121	118–131
5'0"	104–115	113–126	122–137
5'2"	108–121	118–132	128–143
5'4"	114–127	124–138	134–151
5'6"	120–133	130–144	140–159
5'8"	126–139	136–150	146–167
5'10"	132–145	142–156	152–173
6'0"	138–151	148–162	158–179
Men			
5'2"	128–134	131–141	138–150
5'4"	132–138	135–145	142–156
5'6"	136–142	139–151	146–164
5'8"	140–148	145–157	152–172
5'10"	144–154	151–163	158–180
6'0"	149–160	157–170	164–188
6'2"	155–168	164–178	172–197
6'4"	162–176	171–187	181–207